P9-BIB-640

The MACROBIOTIC BROWN RICE COOKBOOK

DELICIOUS AND WHOLESOME GRAIN-BASED DISHES

CRAIG SAMS

Healing Arts Press
Rochester, Vermont

Healing Arts Press
One Park Street
Rochester, Vermont 05767

Copyright 1983, 1988, 1993 by Craig Sams

All rights reserved. No part of this book may be reproduced or utilized in any form or by any means, electronic or mechanical, including photocopying, recording, or by any information storage and retrieval system, without permission in writing from the publisher.

Note to the reader: This book is intended as an informational guide. The remedies, approaches, and techniques described herein are meant to supplement, and not to be a substitute for, professional medical care or treatment. They should not be used to treat a serious ailment without prior consultation with a qualified healthcare professional.

Library of Congress Cataloging-in-Publication Data

Sams, Craig.
    The macrobiotic brown rice cookbook: delicious and wholesome grain-based dishes / Craig Sams.
        p. cm.
    Rev. ed. of: The brown rice cookbook. Rochester, Vt.: Healing Arts Press, 1988.
    Includes index.
    ISBN 0-89281-447-0
    1. Cookery (Brown rice) 2. Macrobiotic diet—Recipes. I. Sams, Craig. The brown rice cookbook. II. Title.
TX809.B75S25 1993
641.6'318—dc20   93-13861
                                                         CIP
Printed and bound in the United States

10 9 8 7 6 5 4 3 2 1

The author wishes to thank Ann Sams for her contribution to the original *Brown Rice Cookbook*, first published in 1981.

Text design by Bonnie Atwater

Healing Arts Press is a division of Inner Traditions International

Distributed to the book trade in the United States by American International Distribution Corporation (AIDC)

Distributed to the book trade in Canada by Publishers Group West (PGW), Montreal West, Quebec

Distributed to the health food trade in Canada by Alive Books, Toronto and Vancouver

CONTENTS

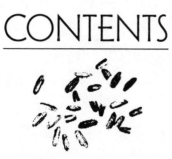

Nature's Perfect Food	1
Macrobiotics in a Nutshell	4
Choosing Your Ingredients	7
Varieties of Rice	15
Cooking Brown Rice	20
Soups	32
Brown Rice and Vegetables	43
Risottos, Casseroles, and Patties	52
Sauces	73
Salads	85
Oriental Rice Dishes	95
Desserts	110
Brown Rice and Fasting	117
Index	121

NATURE'S PERFECT FOOD

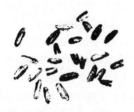

Brown rice is nature's perfect food. As much for its delicious flavor as for its nutritive qualities, it now enjoys widespread popularity, and recent years have seen an enormous increase in the consumption and availability of brown rice. Yet just a few years ago, most available rice was white, and few people even knew what brown rice looked like.

My own love affair with brown rice was triggered by a visit in 1966 to a macrobiotic restaurant called The Paradox, which had recently opened in New York's East Village. Within a year, inspired by its example, I had opened a macrobiotic restaurant in London's Notting Hill. It was a success, and my brother and I went on to open a larger restaurant later that year, called Seed.

The heart of our menu (which we called "Tomorrow's You") was Brown Rice and Vegetables, which sold for four shillings (about 55¢). For hungrier souls, we did a Light Special for seven shillings and sixpence (about $1). The Light Special was usually brown rice and vegetables, with vegetable tempura and a bean dish such as hummus or aduki patties. We also did a Free Meal for those who could not afford these prices. For a while we became the hangout of the "happening scene" of the late sixties, with Terence Stamp, the Beatles, the Rolling Stones, Marc Bolan, and other "faces" of the era regularly dropping in to practice their chopstick technique on a Light Special.

1

By the mid-1970s the bran boom was in full flood, bringing an upsurge in demand for whole wheat bread and pasta, brown rice, and other whole-grain foods. The leading edge of medical research hailed anything with that magic ingredient—dietary fiber—as the cure for all of humankind's ills. Brown rice came in from the cold to become a mainstream food again.

Brown rice is more than just nutritious—it is delicious, with a full, nutty flavor that white rice can never match. It is versatile, enhancing a wide variety of other foods in infinite combinations. How could brown rice once have been almost completely forgotten in favor of white rice? By the 1950s the only devotees were the expanding group of followers in America and Japan who shared macrobiotic pioneer George Ohsawa's interest in traditional nutritional medicine. Ohsawa visited the United States in the 1960s and established a small core of macrobiotic brown rice enthusiasts. From there onward, the consumption of brown rice never looked back. Brown rice has not achieved its preeminence of a few centuries ago, when a few jaded aristocrats in Japan and China were the only consumers of white rice, but it is on its way.

The greatest tragedy of the changeover to white rice is that millions of people whose basic food was rice experienced a quality-of-life deterioration for which the transitory advantages of white rice could never compensate. When we digest carbohydrates, we use up B vitamins. Nature put them in the parts of whole grains that get refined away to make them white. The more white rice one eats, the more B vitamins are needed. If they aren't in the rice or in an accompanying food, the body takes them from its reserves, depriving the brain and other functions of this crucial vitamin group. B vitamin deficiency symptoms include poor coordination, fatigue, apathy, and irritability. No wonder people crave meat in their diets when they consume refined cereal foods—it's the only way they can recover a sense of normality.

White rice may be quick and hassle-free, but few would describe it as better tasting. And it certainly isn't a good source of nutrition. Most of the recipes in this book will work with different varieties of rice or with mixtures of more than one kind. Enjoy.

MACROBIOTICS IN
A NUTSHELL

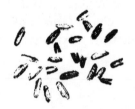

Macro means "big," *bios* means "life." Macrobiotics is the quest to have a big life, in quantity and quality. It's an old word, in use since the seventeenth century, but in modern times it has become associated with Zen macrobiotics, a fusion of traditional Eastern and Western ideas about nutrition and longevity.

Good health is the key to long life and vitality. Health depends on genetic, environmental, and dietary factors. Diet is the factor over which we have most control. A macrobiotic diet is one that is consciously followed with an active awareness of the relation between what you eat and how good you feel. It is a long-term approach to life. It doesn't rule out eating for pleasure, but it also seeks to avoid the painful consequences of eating without understanding.

The study of longevity and of the connection between health and diet has intrigued people since earliest times. The body of knowledge that has come down to us from the past is impressive in its wisdom, and it is free for us to use in creating a macrobiotic way that suits our own particular needs.

Macrobiotics is not a rigid philosophy but a voyage of exploration in which your good judgment is the captain and your body is the ship.

The key principles of macrobiotics today are few and simple:

4

- Eat a diet based on whole grains as the principal food, supplemented by nutrient-rich vegetable foods and seaweeds.
- Maintain a healthy level of physical activity. This means the equivalent of at least half an hour of brisk walking daily.
- Avoid poisons in the environment and in food.
- Consciously maintain a positive mental attitude.
- Practice justice: don't consume more than you need, or through your diet cause unnecessary suffering to other people or to animals.

The diet embodies several specific recommendations:

- Chew food well.
- Minimize the use of nightshades such as tomatoes, potatoes, and eggplant.
- Avoid sugary foods and refined flour products.
- Minimize the use of dairy and animal foods.
- Avoid yeasted foods.
- Eat organically grown food.
- Choose foods that contain no artificial chemicals and that preferably are fresh.
- Avoid alcohol, or use with moderation.

The key to success in macrobiotics is to learn how to cook enjoyable, varied meals using whole-grain and vegetable ingredients. When you surround yourself with good food, it will naturally drive out the bad, and the addictions and cravings that modern diet induces can be kept under control. Eventually the self-discipline you may have to exert at the beginning can wither away as your instincts take over and you enter a virtuous circle of positive development of healthier eating habits. The consciousness change that comes with realizing the direct connection between what you eat and how you feel spills over into the rest of your life.

As long as you fulfill the three conditions for good health—no fatigue, good appetite, and good sleep—the diet and lifestyle you are following is macrobiotic. If you do not fulfill the three conditions, then an understanding of macrobiotic cooking will help you to get there and stay there.

George Ohsawa, the founder of modern macrobiotics, was dismayed at the way people attempted to follow his diet slavishly instead of adapting it to their personal needs. In one of his last books he wrote: "Macrobiotics is a way to build health that enables us to eat and drink *anything we like* whenever we like without being obsessed or driven to do so."

I hope that the recipes in this book help to ensure that you can eat "anything you like" because the food that you like best is good wholesome natural food, cooked for healthy enjoyment.

CHOOSING YOUR INGREDIENTS

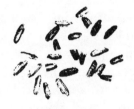

When you have such a well-balanced food as brown rice at the center of your recipes, it is important that you complement it well. Herewith, a few comments about the other ingredients recommended in this book.

BEANS

Brown rice has a balanced protein content, but like other grains is low in one essential amino acid, lysine. Beans and peas contain more lysine in relation to other amino acids. Put them together, and you have a synergistic combination of all the essential amino acids you need. This is seen in the many classic combinations of grains and beans, such as bread with lentil soup, corn tortillas and chili beans, or pita bread and hummus.

Soaking beans for at least 12 hours is a very important aspect of the preparation process: not only are the beans easier to cook to a soft consistency, but in the soaking period the dormant life force of the bean is activated, and it begins the changes that would in a few days lead to sprouting.

This little change makes a great difference to the digestibility and the nutrient availability of the cooked bean—it is no good eating a food because the laboratory analysis shows that it is rich in protein if it gives you indigestion or flatulence and if your digestive system extracts only a small part of the available nutrient content. Never eat raw beans or beans that have not been boiled for at least 10 minutes at full boil before simmering or slow cooking.

Pythagoras, he of the theorem, was a strict vegetarian who would not let his students eat beans because he believed they clouded their reasoning processes. However, this could be because the prevalent bean of ancient Greece was the fava bean—harmless in itself, but with a hard brown skin, which, if regularly eaten, can lead to favism, symptoms of which are deterioration of vision and mental faculties. The Romans, on the other hand, were big fans of beans and named their most famous families after types of beans (Cicero = chick-pea, Fabius = fava).

Aduki beans, chick-peas, lentils, and black beans make ideal complements to brown rice.

VEGETABLES

As with grains and beans, vegetables are much better when organically grown. The advantages of eating foods that do not contain external residues of pesticides or internal traces of systemic herbicides are obvious. Agricultural chemicals are particularly damaging to the body's cleansing organs, like the kidneys and liver. The body doesn't know what to do with them, so it stores the fat-soluble chemicals in an insulating package of fat, in the form of cellulite. This is why the level of pesticides goes up in a person's bloodstream during a diet—the cellulite is breaking down. It takes several generations for the human body to adapt to environmental changes—small consolation if you are exposing yourself to them now. Fortunately, organically grown vegetables, fruits, and grains are increasingly widely available. For the sake of your health—and that of the planet—eat organic, whenever possible.

There are as many different ways to prepare vegetables as there are cooks and knives. The principle to remember is that you want the vegetable pieces to be cooked evenly. The larger you cut a vegetable, the farther the heat has to penetrate before cooking takes place at the core, by which time the outer part has become overcooked. When you cut vegetables in smaller shapes, they cook through quicker and more evenly, and you get more flavor. In stews or casseroles you can cut the vegetables in larger pieces, as the longer cooking time will ensure they are evenly cooked. For stir-fry dishes and quick-cook recipes, keep the pieces smaller and thinner.

SOY FOODS

Meat and dairy products provide distinctive and appealing textures and flavors that are missed when people reduce or exclude them from their diet completely. The humble soybean is a versatile source of alternatives that are more digestible, delicious, and nutritious.

Soy Sauce

Soy sauce is a name that covers a multitude of brown seasonings. At one end of the spectrum is the manufactured soy sauce containing hydrolyzed vegetable proteins, monosodium glutamate, caramel coloring, salt, and water. Real soy sauce or *shoyu* is a naturally fermented product made from a broth of soybeans and wheat, carefully matured together for over a year. Tamari soy sauce is also fermented, from soybeans alone, and has a rich, savory flavor.

Miso Soybean Purée

Miso is a fermented purée made from soybeans and various cereals, using a similar process to naturally made soy sauce. The best ones are fermented for up to 18 months or more. *Genmai miso,* which is made from brown rice and soybeans, has a savory/sweet flavor with a lighter, less bitter taste than some misos.

Soy Milk

A milk can be extracted from soybeans by soaking them in water for a few days, then crushing them in hot water and straining out the milk. Modern processing produces a soy milk that is free from any bitter, "beany" aftertaste and doesn't curdle in hot drinks. It can be used as an alternative to milk in almost all cases but will not set by itself in a pudding the way that milk does.

Tofu

When soy milk is curdled it separates into curds (like cottage cheese) and liquid whey. The curds are then pressed into blocks of tofu, which has a somewhat bland flavor on its own but acts like a sponge in absorbing the flavors of the foods with which it is cooked.

Tempeh

Simply boiled, soybeans lack taste appeal and are not very digestible. When they are fermented for a few days with a specially cultured mold, they bind together to form tempeh, a traditional Indonesian soy food that has a meaty texture and is eminently digestible. Whether it is used in burgers, bacon substitutes, or spreads, tempeh is a versatile and delicious alternative to animal protein.

OILS

Refined oils have no flavor of their own and deteriorate without the addition of antioxidant chemicals. Unrefined oils have distinct flavors, of which olive oil is best known. I use olive oil for sautéing and salads and other lower-temperature uses. Roasted (dark) sesame oil is ideal for stir-frying and other uses where the nutty roasted flavor of the oil complements the other ingredients.

In the fat debate, much is made of which sort of fat one should eat. Far more important is the question of how much you eat. Less is better, when it comes to fat. If you eat too much of *any* kind of fat, whether it is saturated or not, you get fat. Always remove excess fat from foods. Stir-frying is a way of preparing vegetables with a minimum of added fat—keeping the contents of the pan moving keeps them from sticking or burning, and the small amount of oil used captures the flavor of the foods being stir-fried and redistributes it throughout the recipe. Always avoid hydrogenated or partially hydrogenated fats. These are artificially produced from oil that has been chemically altered to make it hard, like plastic. It is a man-made substance that has never existed in nature, and is not, as many people think, simply another saturated oil.

SEAWEEDS AND WILD VEGETABLES

These can, when used in small quantities, provide trace elements that the body needs and that are lacking even in organically grown foods. *Kombu, wakame,* and *arame* from Japan, as well as many indigenous sea vegetables, provide piquant tastes that harmonize with most foods. Green nori flakes are a good way of sprinkling seaweed in sandwiches, soups, mixed vegetable dishes, and pilafs. Not for nothing are nori flakes nicknamed "macrobiotic parsley." Wild vegetables, such as nettles and dandelion leaves, can be used with, or in place of, spinach, where greens are called for. Chickweed is good in salads, and young burdock roots are quite a good substitute for other root vegetables. (They're free, too!) When you gather wild vegetables, make sure that they have not been chemically sprayed—it can sometimes take a few days after spraying before nettles, for example, begin to wilt. If you have a garden, grow your own, and don't worry what the neighbors think!

SEASONINGS

Apart from its usefulness in helping rice to cook to the right texture, salt is often overused in cooking. Because salt affects our overall appetite for food and drink, it is preferable to keep it to a low level that's consistent with good flavor, and let people add more if they need it. Gomasio sesame salt, seaweed and salt blends, soy sauce, or just a salt mill are ways people can add salt at the table. When you adjust the seasoning in a recipe, your tools include soy sauce, salt, bonito flakes, fish sauce, lemon juice, mirin rice wine, plum vinegar, and green nori seaweed flakes, all of which can accent flavors in a recipe. Once you get used to them and learn how they work, you can rely on your instincts to put in a dash of one and a drop of the other to balance the flavors of a recipe.

SEA SALT

Sea salt is preferred because, being unrefined, it contains not only sodium chloride but trace minerals as well. Natural rock crystal salt, which is mined, can be obtained unrefined in health food shops and comes from dried-out prehistoric seas—it has all of the qualities of sea salt.

VEGETABLE STOCK

A good stock makes it much easier to complete the flavor balance in your cooking. Based on *kombu* seaweed and herbs and vegetables of your choice, vegetable stock can be used in all sorts of ways to enhance the flavor of recipes.

SEASONED BREAD CRUMBS
If you have leftover bread, dry it out by gentle baking or in a dry skillet, grate some, and mix the crumbs with salt, herbs, and a little oil. They can then be sprinkled on casseroles (giving a nice crisp top, while keeping the contents moist), used in sauces, and added to soups. Sourdough bread makes particularly flavorful bread crumbs.

DRIED FRUIT
Wherever possible, dried fruit that has not been treated with sulphur dioxide should be used. Raisins are sometimes treated with liquid mineral oil for easier commercial handling, but this is undesirable for domestic use.

SUGAR
Sugar is not included in any of the recipes in this book. In a nutshell, here's why. A healthy appetite is the key to eating a healthy diet. If you repeatedly indulge in foods that unbalance your metabolism, then no amount of brown rice and healthy natural foods can restore the balance. Eating sugar is the fastest way to get your appetite confused, so that you end up having irrational cravings and desperate hunger as your blood sugar goes up to dangerously high levels and then falls to equally dangerous low levels.

Dried fruits, concentrated fruit juices, brown rice syrup, and malt extract all provide slowly metabolized sweetness that does not have the same unbalancing effect on the blood sugar level as cane or beet sugars and glucose.

KITCHEN UTENSILS

All kitchen equipment should be made of nonreactive materials like stainless steel or glass. Aluminum can cause off flavors and colors, enameled pans chip, and cast-iron is best used for frying rather than boiling. The extra investment in stainless-steel utensils is repaid by their longer usable life. If you use a steel wok it should be kept well seasoned and reseasoned if it loses its finish. Use wood, bamboo, or coconut shell utensils when suitable.

FREEDOM

One of the key ingredients of successful cooking is to always do what feels right. Behind your appetite is a complex computer that is constantly examining itself and remembering which foods satisfy which of its requirements. It is presumptuous and arrogant to attempt to be wiser than this experienced intuitive mechanism. All you need are the best natural ingredients and the ability to prepare good food, then let your instincts lead you. Good luck and bon appétit!

VARIETIES
OF RICE

Rice is the principal food crop for half the world's population. It originates from India and Southeast Asia, whence it was brought to Europe by Alexander the Great in 300 B.C. It did not really become a European crop until the Moors introduced it in Spain in the ninth century. It was grown early in United States' colonial history—in South Carolina in 1685—and now is grown mainly in California and the lower Mississippi. In Europe there are three main rice-growing areas—the Po river valley in Lombardy and northern Italy, the Camargue region in the south of France, and the area of Valencia in Spain.

There are two main types of rice, long grain and short grain, but there are many variants within this broad classification. In general, long-grain rices are drier and less sticky. Short-grain rice tends to hold together more and has a stickier texture.

SHORT GRAIN

Short-grain rice grains are about 5 mm (⅕ inch) in length and have a soft texture when cooked. Italian risottos are based on short-grain rices, which have a wide variety of savory uses and are particularly good when served with sauces or with vegetables. Short-grain rice can be served with an ice cream scoop. A more glutinous strain of short-grain rice is found in Japan.

MEDIUM GRAIN

Medium-grain rice is an elongated form of short-grain rice, similar to short-grain but a little longer, about 6 mm (¼ inch). Grown in Italy and the United States, it is mainly refined into white rice.

LONG GRAIN

Long-grain (Indica) rice is slender in shape and can range from 6 to 8 mm (¼ to ⅓ inch) in length. The grains are dry when cooked and barely stick to each other. The best varieties of long-grain rice are grown in subtropical climates, including Thailand, where it is described as "fragrant" rice.

BASMATI RICE

Long-grain rice that is thin and wonderfully aromatic grows in the foothills of the Himalayas. Basmati is the best known of many fine-tasting rices from this region. In Iran there are even more exotic varieties, such as *domsiah* or "royal" rice, *darbori*, and *sadri*, classified in the same way as fine wines. Nowadays, these are disappearing in favor of refined white rice, but the varieties—when you can find them—retain their special flavor.

SWEET BROWN RICE

Sweet brown rice is a very glutinous variety originating from Japan. Its sweet flavor and moist texture when cooked make it ideal for desserts where one wishes to keep sweeteners to a minimum, and also as an addition to some other variety of rice being cooked.

RED RICE

Red rice grows in Southeast Asia and is similar to long-grain in shape. Because it is hardy, it is grown where other rice crops would not thrive. It is dull in color and flavor. Generally the whole grains are eaten by poorer people or used as animal feed.

BLACK RICE

In Southeast Asia a very glutinous blackish-purple rice is widely used. The grains hold together closely when cooked, and the rice is served with stews and soups. It lends itself to eating with the fingers, an old Thai tradition. This rice, as flour, is kneaded with water and forms a strong dough that can be filled and then boiled or steamed.

QUICK RICE

Precooked, re-dried brown rice can be prepared in about 15 minutes and gives a good result. The grains are starchier, and the flavor is sometimes blander, but it certainly saves time, which is people's main complaint about cooking brown rice.

WHITE RICE

Almost any of the above varieties of rice can be turned into white rice by the removal of the bran layers of the grain and the germ to leave the starchy white kernel. The bran and germ contain almost all of the vitamins and minerals and oils of the grain, as well as much of the protein. Not only are nutritive elements lost, but when you eat white rice you eat less fiber. Fiber fills you up and makes you less likely to overeat and gain weight. Fiber also speeds and facilitates the digestive process, for better overall health.

PARBOILED RICE

Also known as "converted rice" and sometimes mistakenly called "brown" rice, this is a processed rice that is the result of an attempt to avoid the worst effects of rice milling. The whole unhusked grains of rice are immersed in hot water and some of the B vitamins and soluble minerals from the bran and germ are absorbed into the starchy white inner part of the grain. The grains are then dried and the bran and germ are removed. The result is a rice that has a dull brown color, little flavor, and just enough B vitamins to keep a frequent consumer from developing beriberi, a B-deficiency disease common where white rice is the staple food.

WILD RICE

Wild rice is not a botanical member of the rice family, but is an aquatic grass whose large, dark grains stand on long stalks in the lakes of Canada and the north central United States. Traditionally harvested by Chippewa Indians, wild rice is no longer any more "wild" than any grain that once upon a time came from a wild plant. After harvest, it is left to ferment in the hull—to increase the flavor and help loosen the hull. It is then lightly toasted, to stabilize the grain. Its high content of lysine, an essential amino acid that is often low in cereals, means that it performs the same role as beans in balancing the amino acid content of a grain-based diet. Use in a proportion of about 5:1 brown rice to wild rice. Its distinctive robust flavor blends well with strong-flavored dishes and piquant sauces.

ABOUT ORGANIC RICE

For extra enjoyment of the recipes in this book, we recommend that you always use organically grown rice. Organically grown food is better nutritionally and is grown using sustainable farming methods that do not deplete the earth's resources or pollute the environment.

In Italy, a large area of the upper reaches of the River Po has come under organic cultivation by a group of organic farmers who realize that modern farming methods threaten to undermine the heritage of the rice paddies that their families have worked for centuries. In rice farming, the decision to grow organically must often be a collective one, as the water is shared by all, and if one farmer uses pesticides, every farm further down the irrigation network gets contaminated. In order to ensure a pure water supply to begin with, the farmers have their water piped from a spring that is fed by melted Alpine snow. The rice grows strong and healthy and is more immune to insects and diseases. Every third year the land is sown in rotation with a cover crop such as alfalfa, to restore fertility. In this way the land is preserved, wildlife has a habitat, and the ability of the land to feed future generations is maintained. As more people choose organic rice, this group of farmers, and the land they cultivate, will expand. These farmers are just one example of responsible stewardship of the countryside that we as consumers must support if we sincerely hope to restore environmental balance and create a sustainable future for the planet.

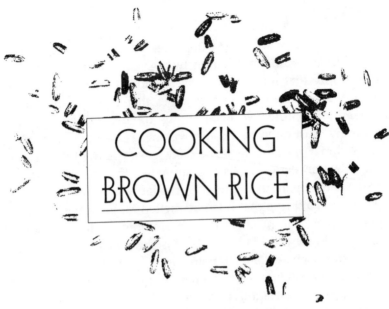

COOKING BROWN RICE

WHAT HAPPENS WHEN BROWN RICE COOKS

The brown rice grain is covered in a layer of bran, permeable to water, but resistant enough to keep the grain from drying out. When the grain is brought to a boil and then reduced to a simmer, the water is absorbed through the bran. It is absorbed into the interior of the grain, softening and moistening every starch cell. Eventually there is no water left between the grains, and the rice is cooked.

Stirring during cooking disturbs this process and breaks the skin of the grains, causing starchiness and stickiness. Once the grains have started to simmer, you should not stir in other ingredients.

Salt plays a role in helping water to pass through the bran and to be absorbed into the grain, so it is always better to add salt before rather than after cooking. If you add too much salt, you may find the grains of rice are a little harder and chewier.

If you add too little salt, they will be softer and starchier. If you want to make salt-free rice, you may find you prefer it if you use slightly less water than recommended in these recipes.

When brown rice is cooked to perfection, you can take some cooked rice between your thumb and forefinger and it will not squash between your fingers nor will pieces fall off. Wait until the rice has cooled a little before doing this!

Always check your rice for the presence of any foreign bodies; a small stone or some other particle can spoil someone's enjoyment of an entire meal. There is no pre-cleaning method that is 100 percent effective, so the extra precaution of picking over your rice is always worth the extra minute or two it may take.

Then, wash your rice. You can simply place the saucepan under a running tap and let the water flow over the top, or shake it in water in an enclosed container and then pour away the water through a strainer. Either way, you get rid of any dust and dirt that may still adhere to the rice.

Boiled Brown Rice

Yield: 4 servings

One of the most important culinary skills you can acquire is to cook brown rice to perfection.

> **3 to 4 cups water***
> **2 cups brown rice**
> **½ teaspoon sea salt**

Bring the water, rice, and salt to a boil in a covered, stainless-steel saucepan. Boil for 3 minutes.

Reduce the heat to the lowest possible level, cover, and simmer for 40 to 60 minutes, or until all of the water has been absorbed and the rice is just beginning to scorch. Do not stir the rice while it is cooking.

Remove the pan from the heat, stir, and let stand for 5 minutes. Then it's ready to serve.

* If you don't use a pan with a tight-fitting or heavy lid, then you will need 3¾ to 4 cups of water to every 2 cups of rice, as more will be lost through evaporation.

Pressure-Cooked Brown Rice

Yield: 4 servings

Because there is less evaporation, you should use less water when pressure-cooking brown rice. This method produces rice of chewier texture than boiled or baked and is ideal when the rice is eaten on its own. Because it holds together better, pressure-cooked brown rice is also more chopstick-friendly.

3 cups brown rice
2 cups water
½ teaspoon sea salt

Bring all of the combined ingredients up to full pressure over medium-high heat. Reduce the heat to low and cook for 35 to 40 minutes.

Remove the pressure cooker from the heat and let stand for at least 10 minutes.

Release the pressure, remove the cover, mix the rice, and serve.

Baked Brown Rice

Yield: 4 servings

This is lighter and fluffier than boiled rice.

2 cups brown rice
3½ cups water
½ teaspoon sea salt

Preheat the oven to 350° F.

For an extra-nutty flavor, stir the rice in a skillet on top of the stove until it is warm and turning a golden brown, about 5 minutes over medium heat.

In a casserole, combine the rice with the water and salt. Cover and bake for 45 minutes, until all the water is absorbed.

Remove, uncover, and allow rice to cool a bit before serving, as it is much hotter straight from the casserole than boiled rice.

Variations

- Add tamari or *shoyu* soy sauce to the rice instead of some of the sea salt.

- A few sautéed vegetables, such as onions or celery, can be added to the rice to infuse it with their flavors.

- Add toasted whole almonds to the rice.

- Add a few pieces of saffron or a pinch of powdered turmeric to the water before it comes to a boil for a yellow color and subtle fragrance.

- If you have a temperature control that will enable you to bake at a low temperature, baked rice can be made overnight, using 3 parts water to 2 parts rice and cooking, tightly covered, at 275° F. This rice is very tasty and chewy; the extra cooking makes it sweeter.

To Reheat Brown Rice

There are various ways to reheat rice that has been cooked earlier:

- *Steaming:* Put the rice in a colander or strainer over a pan of gently boiling water. Cover tightly so that the steam is held by the rice, and cook just until heated through. Remove from the heat before it gets soggy. Uncover and let the rice dry out in the strainer for 1 to 2 minutes before putting it into a serving bowl.
- *Baking:* Heat the rice in a covered container in a preheated 400° F oven for 15 minutes.
- *In pilafs:* If you are adding the rice to other cooked vegetable ingredients, you do not have to preheat it separately. Just stir it, along with cooked ingredients in the pan, to prevent burning. Add a little water to the bottom of the pan to prevent sticking; the rice will be heated as the water evaporates.
- *Microwave:* Place the rice in a nonmetallic dish, cover, and microwave at full power for 2½ minutes.

Steamed Brown Rice

Yield: 4 servings

It is also possible to obtain fluffy rice using the following method. This is particularly recommended for long-grain rice.

1½ **teaspoons sea salt**
4 **cups water**
1½ **cups brown rice, preferably long-grain varieties**

Combine the salt and water and bring to a boil.

Sprinkle the rice into the boiling water. Stir the rice for a moment, cover tightly, and boil gently for 10 to 15 minutes, or until the grains are tender but still brittle in the middle.

Remove the pan from the heat and strain off the water. (Keep it for stock.)

Wrap the partially cooked rice in a linen towel or cheesecloth and steam in a colander or steamer for about 30 minutes, until the rice is fully cooked.

Rice and Wheat

Yield: 4 servings

The combining of different grains adds interest and variety to macrobiotic fare. This recipe is especially good served with Mustard Béchamel Sauce (see page 74).

1 cup wheat (you can also use rye grains)
2 cups brown rice
5 cups water
½ teaspoon sea salt

Presoak the wheat for at least 12 hours in cold water; then drain completely.

Place the wheat, rice, water, and salt in a pressure cooker. Bring the combined ingredients up to full pressure over medium-high heat. Reduce the heat to low and cook for 35 to 40 minutes.

Remove the pressure cooker from the heat and let stand for at least 10 minutes.

Release the pressure, remove the cover, mix, and serve.

Chestnut Rice

Yield: 6 servings

Chestnuts bring a sweet and festive flavor to a meal. They add a richness to rice that is ideal for special occasions and holiday banquets.

1 cup dried, peeled chestnuts
2 cups short-grain brown rice
5½ cups water
½ teaspoon sea salt

Place the chestnuts, rice, water, and salt in a pressure cooker. Bring the combined ingredients up to full pressure over medium-high heat. Reduce the heat to low and cook for 40 minutes.

Remove the pressure cooker from the heat, and let stand for at least 10 minutes.

Release the pressure, remove the cover, mix, and serve.

Traditional
Rice Cream Cereal

Yield: 2 servings

This resulting cereal can be seasoned to taste for a breakfast cereal and is nutritious baby food. It can be puréed with vegetables or fruit for extra flavor.

1 cup cooked brown rice
½ cup water

Purée the cooked rice and extra water and cook to a soft, mushy consistency.

Popped Brown Rice

Popped brown rice is not light and fluffy like popcorn, but it is a deliciously crunchy snack food. The presoaking period enhances the sweetness of the grains. Once you have popped your rice, it can be stored for several weeks in an airtight jar, to be munched as desired.

> **2 cups brown rice**
> **6 cups water, or enough to cover well**
> **3 tablespoons soy sauce**

Combine the rice and water in a bowl. Let stand overnight. Change the water daily for 3 days.

Drain the rice. Heat a skillet, with no oil, over medium heat. Add the drained rice to a depth of ½ inch, and stir constantly until the rice grains dry out, pop, and turn golden brown, about 10 minutes.

Remove the pan from the heat and sprinkle the rice with soy sauce while still hot. Allow to cool completely before storing airtight.

Variation

- Try oven-roasting pumpkin seeds, sesame seeds, or sunflower seeds, and then lightly sprinkle them with natural soy sauce, and mix them with popped rice. You will have a delicious snack that is irresistible, and good for your teeth and gums, if you chew carefully.

Special "Stocks" in Place of Water

Brown rice can be prepared with a variety of liquids. The flavors and colors obtained in this way can subtly enhance the dish in which the rice is used.

The following liquids are good with rice:

- *Vegetable stock:* Use in place of some or all of the water in boiling or baking rice.

- *Tea:* Japanese green tea or twig tea harmonizes well with the flavor of rice.

- *Herb tea:* You can also use various herbal teas that have a distinctive flavor. Try anise, dillseed, tarragon, fennel, or lovage (for a celery-like flavor). If you are going to use the rice cold in a salad, try cooking it with some mint and lemon juice.

- *For rice puddings or when rice is being used in a curry or other spicy dish,* cook brown rice with a few cloves, cinnamon sticks, or coriander seeds to lend a spicy bouquet to the rice.

- *For color,* add a peeled and quartered beet to the water with the rice, and the rice will come out a pinkish color. Saffron or turmeric will give a yellow color. Have fun with nature's food colorings!

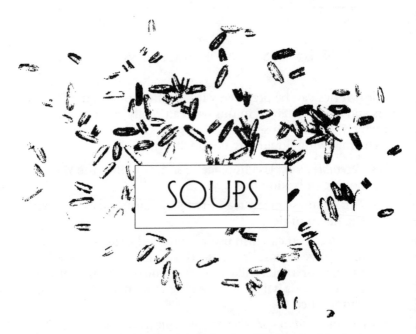

SOUPS

Soup prepares the digestion for food, and sipping hot soup from a spoon somehow evokes that comfortable state of mind in which food should ideally be enjoyed. On a more prosaic level, it moderates the haste with which you attack more substantial food, thereby helping to prevent overeating. When food is eaten quickly, too much can be eaten before the "I'm full now" signal from the stomach reaches the appetite control centers in the brain.

Think in advance about the meal that the soup introduces, and use the soup to contrast and complement the flavors that follow.

Vegetable Stock

Many recipes in this book, especially in this section, call for this Vegetable Stock. If a stock isn't available, water can be substituted. However, a stock brings extra flavor and depth to a recipe.

5 or 6 cups boiling water
1 strip *kombu* seaweed (Leave the white film on the surface of the kombu—this is where some of the flavor comes from.)
Vegetables (This is where the character of the stock develops—see Tips and Variations below.)
Salt, to taste

Boil the water, *kombu,* vegetables, and salt together for a good 30 minutes.
Strain and allow to cool completely.
Refrigerate in a covered jar for up to 5 days.

Tips and Variations
- Celery, fennel, and onions are one good combination.
- Garlic, parsley, and leeks work well.
- Cabbage and broccoli can be too strong tasting if used in excess.
- If you are using organically grown vegetables, then you can use the tops, skins, and otherwise discarded portions of vegetables to build up the stock's flavor.
- Add a few dried shiitake mushrooms, or a handful of fresh mushrooms. (Mushrooms are rich in glutamic acid, a natural protein and flavor enhancer.)
- Don't add fresh stock to old stock. Use up the old stock first,

33

rather than mixing it with fresh stock and then storing it.

- If you have water left over from boiling pasta, use it in place of the water.

- Don't overseason stock—you can always adjust the seasoning in the final recipe. If it is too salty, you can't get the salt out.

- Use fresh herbs where possible, but keep it subtle. Many herbs develop bitter tastes if they are overcooked, so it may be better to add them in your final recipe. However, tarragon, dill, and parsley do not suffer from overcooking. On the other hand, an herb like cilantro (fresh coriander) is best when barely cooked.

Hearty Brown Rice Soup

Yield: 6 servings

The stock is the key to the character of this soup—if you use water then boost the other seasonings.

1 cup chopped onions
1 tablespoon olive oil
1 cup cooked brown rice
Pinch each of thyme, marjoram, and sea salt
½ teaspoon green nori flakes
8 cups boiling vegetable stock or water
1 tablespoon soy sauce
1 cup precooked chick-peas

In a skillet, sauté the onions in oil over medium heat until translucent.

In a large saucepan, combine the onions with all of the remaining ingredients and bring to a boil.

Reduce the heat and simmer for 5 minutes. Serve hot.

Tofu Islands

Yield: 4 servings

Both kudzu *and* arrowroot *act as thickeners and give this soup a consistency similar to stew. They also tend to marry the different flavors in a dish. In the West, arrowroot is by far the more affordable of the two. However,* kudzu *has the additional benefit of easing digestive upsets while soothing and protecting the mucous membrane of the intestinal wall.*

> 1 celery rib, thinly sliced
> 1 carrot, cut into matchsticks
> 4 mushrooms, thinly sliced
> 2 tablespoons olive oil
> 3 cups vegetable stock or water
> 1 cup cooked brown rice
> 1 teaspoon grated fresh ginger
> 1 tablespoon soy sauce
> 2 teaspoons *kudzu* or arrowroot
> 1 cup diced tofu
> Sea salt

In a skillet, sauté the celery, carrots, and mushrooms in the oil until tender, about 5 minutes.

In a large saucepan, combine the stock, rice, ginger, and soy sauce and bring to a boil.

Thoroughly dissolve the *kudzu* in ½ cup water and add it to the boiling stock. When thickened, stir in the vegetables and the tofu; season to taste. Bring back to a boil, and serve hot.

Garlic and Rice Soup

Yield: 2 servings

Try this soup if your taste buds are feeling jaded. It will not only satisfy the most avid garlic lovers, but also clear stuffy heads like magic.

    1 onion, finely chopped
    10 medium garlic cloves, chopped
    3 tablespoons olive oil
    1 cup cooked brown rice
    3 cups vegetable stock or water
    1 tablespoon soy sauce
    ½ cup chopped parsley

In a skillet, sauté the onion and garlic in the oil until golden and turning brown.

In a saucepan, bring the rice, stock, and soy sauce to a boil. Add the onions and garlic and simmer for 10 minutes.

Stir in the parsley just before serving.

Tangy Lemon Soup

Yield: 4 servings

Lemons impart a welcome freshness to hot soups, especially in warm climates. They are popular in the soups of Greece, India, and Morocco.

6 cups vegetable stock
1 cup cooked long-grain brown rice
Juice of 1 lemon
1 cup diced tofu
Sea salt
1 teaspoon grated lemon zest

In a saucepan, bring the stock to a boil. Stir in the cooked rice. Add the lemon juice and tofu and simmer for 10 minutes. Adjust the seasonings (you may find that you will need little or no salt, as lemon juice replaces its flavor contribution).

Add the lemon zest and simmer for another 2 minutes. Serve hot.

Sweet Corn and Rice Soup

Yield: 4 servings

There's no sweet corn like fresh sweet corn in season—use it in this soup if you can.

1 onion, chopped
1 leek, cleaned and sliced crosswise, in rounds
2 tablespoons olive oil
2 cups sweet corn kernels
1 celery rib, sliced
3 cups cooked brown rice
4 cups vegetable stock or water
2 tablespoons soy sauce
Sea salt

In a large saucepan, sauté the onion and leek in the oil until the onions are golden.

Add the corn and celery and stir-fry for 2 minutes.

Add the rice, stock, soy sauce, and sea salt to taste and bring to a boil.

Reduce the heat and simmer gently for 30 minutes.

Adjust the seasonings and serve hot.

Miso Soup with Brown Rice

Yield: 6 servings

Traditionally no Japanese would dream of venturing forth in the morning without a fortifying bowl of miso soup. There are as many ways to prepare miso soup as there are leftover vegetables and grains, but a simple miso broth prepared with the minimum of ingredients can be wonderfully satisfying. The 18-month fermentation period of good-quality miso enables the enzymes to act on the soybeans and grains used to draw out the deepest and subtlest components of flavor. It is hard to believe that this flavorful food can be the transformation of such bland ingredients. That's the wonder of enzymes!

The following recipe uses the mellow-flavored genmai *miso, which is made from brown rice and soybeans.*

1 onion, chopped
2 tablespoons roasted (dark) sesame oil
1 carrot, cut into matchsticks
1 cup bean sprouts
7 cups boiling vegetable stock or water
2 cups cooked brown rice
½ cup **genmai miso**

In a large saucepan, sauté the onions in the oil until translucent, about 5 minutes. Add the carrot and bean sprouts and sauté for 3 to 5 minutes more.

Add the boiling stock and rice to the vegetables and simmer for a further 5 minutes.

Combine the miso with 1 cup cold water and mix thoroughly. Add the mixture to the soup, bring just to a boil, and serve hot.

Variations

- Add a few strips of *wakame* seaweed to the stock before bringing it to a boil.
- Add 2 teaspoons lemon juice and 1 tablespoon rice syrup or apple juice concentrate to get a more sweet-sour taste.

Nettle Soup

Yield: 4 servings

Whenever using wild vegetables, make sure that they are not from an area that has recently been sprayed with herbicides. Gather stinging nettles with rubber gloves and a generous-sized bag—they take up a lot of space.

1 pound stinging nettles
1 onion, chopped
2 garlic cloves, sliced
2 tablespoons olive oil
6 cups boiling vegetable stock or water
1 cup cooked brown rice
1 tablespoon lemon juice
Sea salt
1 teaspoon black pepper

Wearing gloves, remove the tops and tender young leaves of the nettles and discard the stalks. Chop lightly.

In a large saucepan, sauté the onion and garlic in the oil until golden. Add the nettles and stir-fry for several minutes—until the nettles have shrunk to a quarter of their original volume.

Add the boiling stock to the nettle and onion mixture. Stir in the rice, lemon juice, and seasonings, and simmer for 10 minutes before serving.

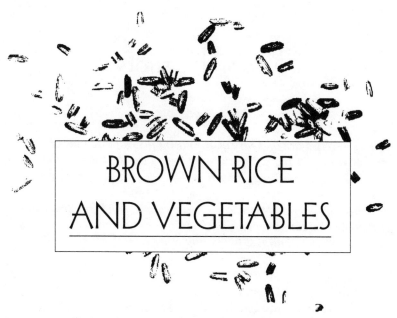

BROWN RICE
AND VEGETABLES

This classic dish, in all its variations, serves as the all-in-one vegetarian, macrobiotic, gluten-free, yeast-free, organic staple meal. Despite the limitations implied by its title, the permutations are infinite. In his reflections on his childhood days, Mao Tse Tung never seemed to be aware of the advantages of brown rice and vegetables in the diet. His father, an ambitious farmer, turned his livestock into cash at the local market, and restricted young Mao and the family to a less rich and more wholesome diet of brown rice and vegetables. While the diet probably laid the foundations for his strong constitution and longevity, who knows what resentment of the profit motive developed in his mind as he watched the live produce of his father's farm being trotted off to grace richer folks' tables?

Rice and Carrots

Yield: 4 servings

This is a very quick and easy dish. When I first got into macrobiotics, this was almost my entire culinary repertoire. As my horizons expanded, I left it behind, only to rediscover it happily many years later.

If you are not using organically grown carrots, peel them thoroughly, as commercial carrot-growing methods involve saturating the soil with more insecticide than just about any other vegetable.

3 tablespoons sesame seeds
3 medium-large carrots, coarsely grated
3 tablespoons roasted (dark) sesame oil
3 cups cooked brown rice

In a dry, stainless-steel skillet, toast sesame seeds over medium heat until golden and fragrant, about 10 minutes. Stir frequently to prevent scorching.

In a saucepan or large skillet, sauté the carrots in the oil for 4 to 5 minutes, until just soft. Add the sesame seeds and mix well. Stir in the brown rice and ¼ cup water. Cover, and cook over gentle heat until the water is absorbed, about 5 minutes.

Serve immediately.

Mushrooms and Rice

Yield: 2 servings

The "meaty" texture of mushrooms is a wonderful addition to grain and vegetable dishes. Try different varieties of mushroom for their distinctive and delicate flavors.

1 onion, chopped
3 tablespoons vegetable oil
1½ cups sliced mushrooms
3 cups cooked long-grain brown rice
2 tablespoons soy sauce

Garnish
Chopped parsley

In a skillet, sauté the onion in the oil until translucent, about 4 minutes. Add the mushrooms and sauté until the mushrooms are tender and cooked through, about 7 minutes.

Stir in the rice, soy sauce, and 3 tablespoons of water. Cover and simmer gently over low heat until the water is absorbed, about 3 minutes.

Serve right away, garnished with chopped parsley.

Variations

- Add garlic to enhance the mushroom flavor.
- Use presoaked or fresh shiitake mushrooms, sliced into strips.

Aduki Rice

Yield: 4 servings

There are two ways to enjoy the synergy of aduki beans and brown rice. One way is simply to substitute presoaked aduki beans for some of the brown rice when cooking the rice. The water absorption and the cooking time are the same for adukis and brown rice. Wash and presoak the adukis overnight for best results. The kombu *helps soften the beans.*

½ teaspoon sea salt
5 cups water
1 cup dried aduki beans
2 cups brown rice
1 strip *kombu* seaweed

In a large saucepan or skillet, combine the sea salt and water and bring to a boil.

Add the aduki beans and rice and bring back to a boil.

Reduce the heat to a simmer, and add the *kombu*. Cover, and cook for 35 to 45 minutes, or until the water is absorbed. Serve immediately.

Rice and Peas

Yield: 2 servings

This traditional combination of complementary proteins is the nutritional mainstay of the Caribbean people. They use gungo peas (cow peas) or red kidney beans in the role of the bean in this simple recipe. I prefer it with adukis and have left it to you to add the scorching red peppers that are often a feature of this recipe.

1 cup cooked adukis
3 cups cooked brown rice
½ cup vegetable stock
½ cup unsweetened coconut milk
Sea salt
Pepper

In a saucepan, combine all of the ingredients and bring to a boil. Reduce the heat and simmer for 5 minutes, or until the liquid has been absorbed.

Serve immediately.

Belizian Brown Rice Mix-it-up

Yield: 2 to 3 servings

Some years ago my cousin Tony, who was in Belize filming the Maya Deer Dance in celebration of the Harmonic Convergence (a crucial date in the Mayan calendar), asked me to come along and help carry the cameras.

We set up headquarters in the southernmost town, Punta Gorda, population 2,000. It is the capital city of the remote southern Toledo district, mostly inhabited by the Mayans. The locals call it "the forgotten district," and with no banks or taxis, it is primitive. The guest house we stayed in wasn't quite ready to open, but it was the only place in town. The owner, Chet Schmidt, was an American, harboring a dream of bringing eco-tourists to the Toledo district.

We got to talking one evening, and he reminisced about his early days, mentioning that he had opened the first macrobiotic restaurant on the West Coast, on Telegraph Avenue in Berkeley in mid-1967. Even more astonishing, he had also been inspired to do so by a visit to The Paradox restaurant in New York's East Village in mid-1966. We compared notes and realized that we each had taken exactly a year from visiting The Paradox to opening the restaurant that our visit there inspired; his was 3,000 miles west in Berkeley, and mine was 3,000 miles east in London.

This recipe is based on the food that became our staple fare in Belize, picked straight from his fruit and vegetable garden. If you can't get plantains, then use bananas.

    4 plantains, each sliced lengthwise into 4 long slices
    6 tablespoons vegetable oil
    Sea salt
    2 onions, chopped

3 cups cooked long-grain brown rice
½ cup unsweetened coconut milk
Ground cinnamon
Pepper

In a skillet, fry the plantains in 3 tablespoons of the vegetable oil, sprinkling lightly with salt, and turning when the underside has just started to brown; set aside.

Sauté the onions in the remaining oil until soft. Stir in the brown rice, coconut milk, and cinnamon and pepper to taste. Simmer over low heat until the liquid has been absorbed, about 5 minutes.

Arrange the rice and onion mixture in the center of a plate, and cover with the fried plantain slices. Serve at once.

Rice and Greens

Yield: 2 to 3 servings

Green vegetables are rich in vitamin A, boost the immune system, and also help prevent anemia. There are all sorts of greens you can use—we freely use (and mix) cabbage greens, kale, collard greens, arugula leaves. You can also use dandelion leaves, cauliflower leaves, radicchio, curly endive, and flat parsley leaves.

1 onion, halved and sliced
2 garlic cloves, chopped
8 scallions, sliced
3 tablespoons roasted (dark) sesame oil
1 pound greens, sliced into strips

1 teaspoon chopped fresh ginger
3 cups cooked brown rice
1 teaspoon grated lemon zest
1 teaspoon lemon juice
Soy sauce
Sea salt

In a saucepan, sauté the onion, garlic, and scallions in the oil for 4 minutes. Add the greens and ginger and stir-fry for another few minutes, until soft.

Stir in the rice, lemon zest, and lemon juice, and combine well. Season to taste with soy sauce and salt.

Add enough water to cover the bottom of the pan (less than ¼ inch). Cover the pan, and simmer gently until water is absorbed, about 5 minutes. Serve immediately.

Variation

• Add herbs generously to this recipe—fresh marjoram goes well, try fresh dill or fennel, sprinkle Japanese wasabi horseradish powder in to give it more bite.

Tarragon Rice and Peas

Yield: 2 to 3 servings

This recipe was originally a Tarragon Kedgeree, a rice dish based on flaked white fish and tarragon. However, whether you make it with fish, tofu, or as per the recipe below, the flavor of the tarragon is the key ingredient. Tarragon doesn't dry well—if you can't get fresh, use freeze-dried, and reconstitute with water for 20 minutes before using. You can use snow peas or frozen peas—you don't need to thaw them out.

2 onions, chopped
4 garlic cloves, chopped
2 tablespoons olive oil
1 cup green peas or whole snow peas
¼ cup lightly chopped fresh tarragon leaves
3 cups cooked brown rice
Vegetable stock or water

Garnish
1 lemon, quartered

In a large skillet, sauté the onions and garlic in the olive oil until translucent, about 5 minutes.

Add the peas, tarragon, and rice and combine well. Add just enough vegetable stock or water to barely cover the bottom of the pan. Cover and simmer for a few minutes until the water is absorbed.

Serve right away, garnished with lemon quarters.

51

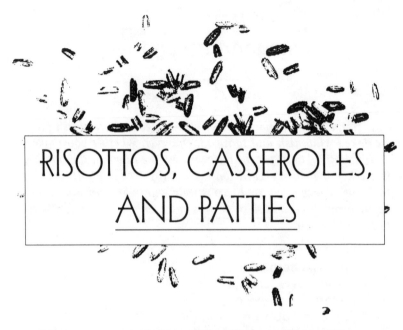

RISOTTOS, CASSEROLES, AND PATTIES

Often rice is cooked along with other ingredients. These cooking methods usually apply when white rice is used because the long cooking time of brown rice means that by the time the rice is done, everything else is overcooked. However, the recipes that follow work equally well with brown rice, infusing the rice grains with the flavors of the other ingredients.

Autumn Risotto

Yield: 4 servings

The vegetables in this recipe are especially flavorful when they are fresh from the garden. It's worth the trouble to obtain them this way in late summer and autumn when home gardeners have an abundance. Organically grown and fresh, these humble vegetables acquire noble status in this recipe.

¼ cup plus 1 tablespoon olive oil
1 onion, chopped
2 carrots, diced
3 zucchinis, cut into broad matchsticks
1 cup shredded cabbage
2½ cups short-grain brown rice
5 cups vegetable stock or water
3 garlic cloves, crushed
Sea salt
¼ teaspoon black pepper
3 tablespoons chopped parsley

Preheat the oven to 350° F.

Heat the oil in a heavy casserole. Add all of the vegetables and cook, stirring constantly, until they begin to soften, about 5 minutes.

Add the rice and stir for 2 to 3 minutes. Stir in the stock. Add the garlic and parsley and season with the salt and pepper. Bring the mixture to a boil. Transfer the casserole, uncovered, to the oven and bake for 35 minutes.

Remove from the oven and let stand for 10 minutes before serving.

Tempeh Casserole

Yield: 3 to 4 servings

As a child my mother taught me how to make sugary cakes and cookies, skills that have subsequently been of little value. However, her casserole recipe has been a mainstay of my cooking for decades. Thanks, Mom!

Sauce

1 onion, chopped
3 garlic cloves, chopped
¼ cup olive oil
¼ cup plus 1 tablespoon whole wheat flour
1½ cups vegetable stock or water
1 tablespoon soy sauce
½ teaspoon sea salt

Filling

1 onion, chopped
2 tablespoons olive oil
1 cup cubed tempeh
3 cups cooked brown rice
2 cups fresh or frozen green peas
1 cup seasoned bread crumbs (see page 13)

Preheat the oven to 350° F.

To make the sauce: In a saucepan, sauté the onion and garlic in the oil, until golden.

Add the flour and stir-fry over low heat for 3 to 4 minutes, making sure not to let the flour burn.

Slowly add the stock, stirring constantly to ensure lumps do not form. Cook until the sauce thickens, about 3 minutes. Add soy sauce and salt to taste. Set aside.

To make the filling: In a skillet, sauté the onion in the olive oil until golden.

Add the reserved sauce along with the tempeh, rice, and peas. Fold together well. The sauce should be runny enough to coat every grain of rice and bind everything together.

Place the mixture in a casserole dish and sprinkle evenly with the seasoned bread crumbs. Cover and bake for 30 minutes, until the crumbs are browned. Let cool for 5 minutes before serving.

Note: This basic concept—of mixing a mock béchamel sauce with rice and vegetables, covering, and baking it—has infinite permutations. It can be made with fish, such as tuna, it can be made with tofu, and it can be made with other vegetables as well as peas.

Risi i Bisi

Yield: 4 servings

This is the traditional dish of Italy's Veneto region, which includes Venice. Our version doesn't contain ham or Parmesan cheese.

1 onion, chopped
2 tablespoons olive oil
1 pound shelled (fresh or frozen) green peas
3 cups vegetable stock or water
1 cup soy milk
2 cups short-grain rice
¼ teaspoon sea salt

In a saucepan, sauté the chopped onion in the oil until golden. Add the peas and stir-fry for 2 minutes. Add the stock and the soy milk and bring to a boil.

When the mixture is bubbling, stir in the rice and the salt. Cover, reduce the heat to low, and simmer gently, stirring every 10 minutes, until the rice has absorbed most of the liquid. The center of the rice should still be slightly crunchy—that's the Italian way—while the sauce should still be wet, but not soupy. You should be able to pick it up on a fork without dripping. Feel free to add more liquid, and cook further, if you think it is too dry.

Remove from the heat and serve immediately.

Cashew Risotto

Yield: 2 servings

Roasted cashews transform this dish, giving it a rich and elegant flavor.

1 cup raw or roasted cashew nuts
Grated zest and juice of 1 lemon
3 cups cooked brown rice
1 cup cubed tofu
2 tablespoons chopped parsley
Soy sauce
Sea salt
Pinch of ground cinnamon
Seasoned whole wheat bread crumbs

If the cashews are raw, toast them in a shallow dish for 20 minutes in a 325° F oven.

Preheat the oven to 300° F. Oil a casserole or baking dish.

In a bowl, combine the cashews, lemon zest, lemon juice, brown rice, tofu, and parsley. Season with soy sauce, salt, and cinnamon to taste.

Place the mixture in the oiled baking dish. Sprinkle the top with the seasoned bread crumbs ¼ inch deep. Bake for 20 to 25 minutes, until the top is lightly browned. Serve immediately.

Spring Risotto

Yield: 3 servings

Harvesting your own dandelion greens in the springtime adds adventure and satisfaction to this recipe.

1 onion, chopped
2 leeks, cleaned and sliced crosswise, in rounds
¼ cup plus 1 tablespoon olive oil
1 pound broccoli, cut into florets
2 cups chopped greens (cabbage, dandelion leaves, mustard greens)
3 cups cooked long-grain brown rice
Sea salt
Black pepper
½ cup vegetable stock or water

Garnish
4 scallions, finely chopped

In a saucepan, sauté the onion and leeks in the oil until the onions are translucent, about 5 minutes.

Add the broccoli and greens, and stir-fry for 3 to 4 minutes, until just tender.

Stir in the brown rice and season with salt and pepper to taste.

Pour the stock over the contents, cover, and simmer gently until the stock has been absorbed, about 5 minutes.

Sprinkle with the scallions and serve at once.

Sunshine Risotto

Yield: 4 servings

This delicious dish combines the nuttiness of toasted seeds with the sweetness of dried fruits to give an exotic flavor and a satisfying meal. Traditional "one pot" cuisine puts all the tastes into one dish—sweet, sour, salty, bitter, pungent, and spicy.

1 cup sunflower seeds
2 tablespoons flaxseeds
1 carrot, diced
2 onions, chopped
3 celery ribs, chopped
2 tablespoons vegetable oil
3 cups cooked brown rice
½ cup raisins
½ cup currants
½ cup vegetable stock or water
1 teaspoon soy sauce
½ teaspoon sea salt

Combine the seeds on a baking sheet and toast in a 350°F oven for 7 to 8 minutes. Leave the oven on.

In a skillet, sauté the carrot, onions, and celery in the oil until the onions are translucent.

Sprinkle the seeds over the vegetables. Stir in the rice, raisins, currants, stock, sea salt, and soy sauce.

Transfer the mixture to a medium-sized casserole. Cover and bake for 15 minutes, until the top is lightly browned. Serve immediately.

Risoverde

Yield: 3 servings

Elizabeth David, the late lamented doyenne of food writers, who singlehandedly dragged English cuisine away from meat, potatoes, and boiled vegetables toward an understanding of Mediterranean food styles, includes this recipe in her 1954 book, Italian Food. *The recipe's origins are quoted as "Marinetti—La Cucina Futurista" (Futuristic Cooking).*

1 onion, chopped
2 tablespoons olive oil
1 pound mixed greens (mustard, spinach, or radicchio),
  chopped
Sea salt
1 cup vegetable stock or water
1 cup green peas, cooked until soft
½ cup shelled pistachio nuts
3 cups cooked brown rice

In a saucepan, sauté the onion in the oil until golden. Add the greens and salt and stir-fry over high heat for 3 minutes.

Add the stock, cover, and simmer gently until the stock is absorbed and the greens are tender.

Purée the green peas with the pistachios to make a thick cream. Add a little water, if necessary.

Heat the rice and serve on a bed of the cooked greens, covered with the pea and pistachio purée.

Risotto in Salto

**Yield: variable, depending on how much
cooked rice you have in the refrigerator**

*For any leftover rice pilaf, risotto, or just plain rice, this is a great
snack or appetizer.*

**Leftover rice or risotto
Seasoned bread crumbs (page 13)
Olive oil
Chopped parsley
Soy sauce**

Form the rice into large flat patties and coat with the seasoned
bread crumbs.

Gently fry the patties in the oil over low heat until well
cooked. Remove from pan and serve, sprinkled with chopped
parsley and soy sauce.

Stuffed Vine Leaves

Yield: 4 servings

When immigrants from Greece and the Middle East came to the United States they couldn't believe their luck—grape leaves grew wild everywhere, free for the picking, and all spring and summer long. Normally grape leaves are an occasional delicacy, as they are needed by the grapevine to fulfill vital photosynthesis activities. However, the wild grapes that tumble down river banks and thrive in the northeastern United States are an ideal substitute for the larger leaves of their European cousin, Vitis vinifera.

If you harvest them, keep an eye peeled for poison ivy—I once harvested some by accident just after twilight near Doylestown, Pennsylvania, only discovering my mistake when I tipped out my bag on the kitchen table.

1 onion, chopped
6 garlic cloves, chopped
2 tablespoons olive oil
3 cups cooked brown rice
½ cup pine nuts
1 tablespoon green nori flakes (optional)
Sea salt
About 20 grape leaves
1 cup vegetable stock or water
1 tablespoon soy sauce

Preheat the oven to 350° F. Oil a medium-sized casserole or baking dish.

In a skillet, sauté the onion and garlic in the oil until lightly browned, 5 to 6 minutes.

62

Add the brown rice, pine nuts, nori, and salt; set aside.

Cook the grape leaves in boiling salted water for 2 to 3 minutes; drain and allow to cool.

Place 1 tablespoonful of the rice mixture on each leaf, and roll up, tucking in the ends as soon as one complete turn is made. Place the rolls side by side in the prepared dish. Pour the stock and soy sauce over the rolls.

Cover and bake for 25 minutes. Serve immediately.

Note: Stuffed vine leaves can be enjoyed hot or cold served cold; they are good with a wedge of lemon.

Cabbage Rolls

Yield: 4 servings

This traditional dish (vegetarian style) can be enjoyed hot or cold, and is especially good with sweet and sour dipping sauce.

2 onions, chopped
6 garlic cloves, chopped
2 tablespoons olive oil
3 cups cooked brown rice
Sea salt
1 green cabbage, cored but left whole
1 cup vegetable stock, cabbage cooking liquid, or water

Preheat the oven to 350° F.

In a skillet, sauté the onions and garlic in the oil until lightly browned, 5 to 6 minutes.

Combine the mixture with the brown rice and sea salt to taste. Set aside.

Boil the head of cabbage in salted water to cover for 5 to 7 minutes until the leaves are tender. Remove from the water, drain, and allow to cool. Peel off the outer leaves slowly, taking care not to tear them.

Place 3 tablespoonfuls of the rice mixture on each leaf, and roll up, tucking in the ends as soon as one complete turn is made. Place the rolls side by side in an oiled casserole or baking dish.

Pour the stock over the cabbage rolls. Cover and bake for 25 minutes. Serve immediately.

Peanut Rice Supreme

Yield: 4 servings

Peanuts and peanut butter always have a special appeal for chil-dren, but adults will also appreciate the subtle and delicious flavor of this recipe.

1 onion, chopped
1 cup chopped celery
3 tablespoons roasted (dark) sesame oil
1 cup roasted, coarsely chopped peanuts
3 cups cooked brown rice
1 cup cubed tofu
½ cup peanut butter
1 tablespoon soy sauce
½ teaspoon sea salt
½ cup whole wheat bread crumbs
½ cup vegetable stock or water

Preheat the oven to 375° F. Liberally oil a medium-sized casserole.

In a skillet, sauté the onion and celery in the oil until the onions are golden. Add all of the remaining ingredients and mix together well. You should be able to form it in your hands.

Place the mixture in the prepared casserole and pat down.

Cover and bake for 30 to 40 minutes, or until the top is browned.

Remove from the oven, and let cool for a few minutes. Unmold onto a serving platter.

Stuffed Onions

Simmering, sautéing, and baking combine in this recipe to bring out the natural sweetness and delicate flavor of onions.

4 large onions, peeled
3 tablespoons olive oil
1 cup chopped mushrooms
2 cups cooked brown rice
½ cup seasoned bread crumbs (page 13)
1 tablespoon soy sauce
½ teaspoon fresh or dried thyme
¼ teaspoon black pepper
½ teaspoon sea salt

Simmer the onions in boiling water until tender, at least 30 minutes. Drain and set aside to cool.

Preheat the oven to 350° F.

Slice off the onion tops and remove the centers with a spoon, leaving onion shells that can be filled.

Chop the onion centers.

In a skillet, sauté the chopped onion centers in the oil with the mushrooms for 5 minutes, or until the mushrooms soften.

Stir in all of the remaining ingredients and mix well.

Pour ½ inch of water into a casserole. Fill the onion shells with the stuffing mixture, and place side by side in the casserole dish.

Cover and bake for 30 to 45 minutes, or until the onions are golden.

Stuffed Summer Squash

Yield: 4 servings

The roasted buckwheat in this recipe provides a light texture and a hearty, nutty flavor.

1 medium summer squash
1 onion, finely chopped
3 garlic cloves, finely chopped
2 tablespoons vegetable oil
2 cups cooked brown rice
1 cup cooked roasted buckwheat*
¾ cup chopped roasted hazelnuts (filberts)
1 teaspoon fresh or dried marjoram
½ teaspoon sea salt
1 teaspoon black pepper
1 cup vegetable stock or water

Preheat the oven to 375° F.

Cut the squash lengthwise in half and scoop out the seeds. Lay the halves side by side in a baking dish.

In a skillet, sauté the onion and garlic in the oil until light golden.

Combine the onion and garlic with all of the remaining ingredients and mix well.

Spoon the mixture into the hollowed-out halves of squash. Pour ½ cup water into the bottom of the dish. Cover, and bake for 45 minutes, or until the squash is cooked through. Serve right away.

*To cook roasted buckwheat, pour 2 parts boiling water over 1 part buckwheat. Simmer for 10 minutes over low heat. Let stand for 10 minutes in a covered saucepan.

Brown Rice Tray *Kibbeh*

Yield: 6 servings

*This traditional Middle Eastern dish is baked in a flat pan, or "tray."
It is usually made with bulgur wheat, which is whole wheat that
has been cooked, dried, and then cracked. It therefore absorbs water when soaked, and has a sweeter taste than raw whole wheat. If
my Syrian grandmother were alive I hate to think what she would
say about my making this recipe with brown rice. She would probably be so shocked that a man of the family was deeply involved in
cooking* kibbeh *that she wouldn't even notice the brown rice!*

Shell
1 medium onion, finely
  chopped
2 cups soaked bulgur wheat
2 cups cooked brown rice
1½ cups *seitan* (wheat
  gluten), chopped
1 teaspoon sea salt
1 teaspoon black pepper
½ teaspoon ground cin-
  namon
½ teaspoon ground allspice

Filling
1 onion, chopped
3 garlic cloves, chopped
2 tablespoons olive oil
1½ cups pine nuts
3 tablespoons chopped
  parsley
1 teaspoon sea salt
1 teaspoon black pepper
1 teaspoon ground cinnamon

To make the shell: Preheat the oven to 375° F. Oil a shallow
8- by 12-inch pan.

Although traditionally the shell should be made in a mortar
with a pestle, I prefer a food processor! Mix together all of the
ingredients for the shell in a bowl. (Do not cook the onion.)

Add a small amount of the mixture into the food processor at a time. Process until the mixture holds together when you form it in your hands. Add water, if needed, or add a little whole wheat flour to dry the mixture out. Set aside.

To make the filling: In a skillet, sauté the onion and garlic in the oil until light golden. Add the pine nuts and stir-fry until the pine nuts start to turn brown. Add the parsley, salt, pepper, and cinnamon. Set aside.

Pat half of the shell mixture in an even layer over the bottom of the pan. Cover with all of the filling. Pat the remaining shell mixture on top of the filling. Pierce with a fork. Brush lightly with oil.

Bake for 30 minutes.

Slice the *kibbeh* as soon as you remove it from the oven. Let cool for 10 minutes before serving.

Brown Rice Patties

Yield: 4 servings (8 patties)

This is a delicious way of using leftover rice, and surplus patties can be kept refrigerated or frozen for later use.

1 cup chopped onion
1 tablespoon olive oil
3 cups cooked brown rice
¼ cup finely chopped parsley
½ cup roasted sunflower seeds
3 scallions, chopped
Pinch of sea salt
1 cup Mock Béchamel Sauce (page 74)
Whole wheat flour
Vegetable oil, for frying

In a skillet, sauté the onion in the oil until golden, about 5 minutes.

In a bowl, combine the onions, rice, parsley, sunflower seeds, scallions, salt, and mock béchamel sauce. Mix to bind the ingredients together.

Shape the mixture into patties, and dust with the flour.

Pour ¼ inch of vegetable oil into a skillet. Fry the patties, turning once, until browned on both sides. Serve at once.

Bean Sprout and Rice Patties

Yield: 4 servings (8 patties)

Sprouts are bursting with life and essential nutrients. They add a lightness and "crunch" to rice patties.

1 onion, chopped
1 tablespoon olive oil
3 cups cooked brown rice
½ cup toasted sunflower seeds
1 cup bean sprouts
¼ cup finely chopped parsley
½ cup whole wheat bread crumbs
Oat flakes (to cover)
Vegetable oil, for frying

In a skillet, sauté the onion in oil until translucent.

In a bowl, combine the onion, rice, sunflower seeds, sprouts, parsley, and bread crumbs. Form the mixture into 3-inch-long sausage shapes. Roll each one in oats flakes.

Pan-fry in ½ inch of oil, turning once, about 5 minutes each side. Serve immediately or leave to cool—the patties are delicious cold, too.

Brown Rice and Peanut Butter Bake

Yield: 4 servings

This recipe goes down well with children as a treat. The cooked slices travel easily for picnics and in lunch boxes.

8 ounces tofu
3 cups cooked brown rice
¾ cup crunchy peanut butter
1 onion, chopped and sautéed
1 tablespoon sugar-free ketchup

Preheat the oven to 350° F. Oil a loaf pan.

Crumble the tofu into a mixing bowl. Add all of the other ingredients and mix well.

Place the mixture in the prepared pan. Bake for 40 to 50 minutes, until the top is browned.

When done, let cool for a few minutes, turn upside down, and the loaf should fall away intact. You can serve this hot or cold.

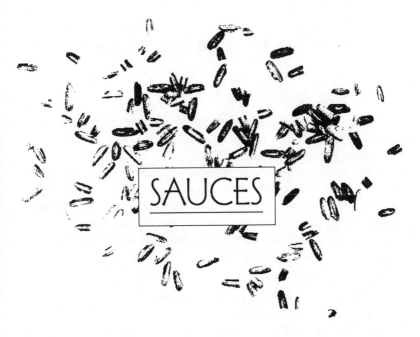

SAUCES

Sometimes brown rice with an appropriate sauce can make a complete meal. The sauce is an enhancer to the brown rice, rather than an accompaniment. It gives a character to brown rice that harmonizes it with the other parts of the meal.

Mock Béchamel Sauce

Yield: 4 servings

This recipe comes originally from Zen Cookery—the first English-language macrobiotic cookbook, published in 1965. When I first discovered béchamel sauce it added a whole new dimension to eating rice. With the sweetness of onions, a hint of garlic, and well-toasted flour, it complements the texture and flavor of brown rice perfectly. When you toast flour and then cook it with water, the complex starches break down into simpler starches called malto-dextrins. Their sweetness is subtle at first, but as you chew, it becomes more pronounced.

1 onion, finely chopped
2 garlic cloves, chopped
¼ cup olive oil
¼ cup plus 1 tablespoon whole wheat flour
1½ cups water or vegetable stock
Soy sauce
Sea salt

In a skillet, sauté the onion and garlic in the oil until translucent.

Add the flour, mix well, and stir while frying for another 3 minutes, taking care that it does not burn.

Slowly add the water, stirring constantly to prevent lumps, until the sauce thickens. Season to taste with soy sauce and sea salt.

Variations

- Mustard Béchamel—Add 2 teaspoons mustard or 1 teaspoon mustard powder and 1 tablespoon lemon juice to the sauce.

- Wasabi Béchamel—Put a teaspoon or two of wasabi powder in the sauce in place of mustard for an even more pungent flavor.
- Dill and Pea Béchamel—Add 2 teaspoons chopped dill leaves and ½ cup thawed frozen peas to the completed sauce.
- Increasing the oil content makes for a creamier, richer sauce.

Almond Sauce

Yield: 4 servings

Ground nuts give extra body to sauces and harmonize well with rice. Use almonds roasted or raw with equally good results.

½ cup ground almonds
2 cups vegetable stock
2 garlic cloves, chopped
2 tablespoons chopped parsley
Juice of 1 lemon
Sea salt
Pinch of black pepper
Pinch of ground cinnamon (optional)

Garnish
Chopped nuts or herbs

In a saucepan, mix all of the ingredients together, seasoning to taste. Simmer gently until the sauce thickens, about 20 minutes.

Serve over rice, sprinkled with chopped nuts or herbs.

Vegetable Sauce

Yield: 4 servings

You can choose different vegetables for this recipe, depending on what is available, to achieve an infinite number of variations.

1 onion, thinly sliced
3 garlic cloves, chopped
1 carrot, grated
3 tablespoons vegetable oil
1 cup vegetable stock or water
3 tablespoons soy sauce
2 teaspoons freshly grated ginger
1½ tablespoons *kudzu*, dissolved in ½ cup cold water

In a skillet, sauté the onion, garlic, and carrot in the oil until they are tender, about 5 minutes.

Add the stock, soy sauce, and ginger and bring to a boil. Simmer gently for 3 minutes.

Add the *kudzu* and water mixture and stir constantly until the sauce thickens and is translucent.

Variation

• You can use almost any vegetable combination for this sauce. The key is to keep the pieces small, but still distinct. If you use bean sprouts in this sauce, use them whole; they will give the sauce texture. Peas or sweet corn kernels should also be used whole. Of course, if you have leftover vegetables strained from the vegetable stock, a sauce like the above is a useful way to use them. Reduce the cooking time for them, as they have already been well cooked in making the stock.

Sweet and Sour Sauce

Yield: 4 servings

This sauce is good when you serve brown rice with fried foods such as tempura or satay-style kebabs of tofu or tempeh.

1 tablespoon sesame oil
1 onion, thinly sliced
1 carrot, finely diced
1 cup vegetable stock or water
2 tablespoons soy sauce
3 tablespoons apple juice concentrate
1 tablespoon vinegar (brown rice or apple cider)
Sea salt
2 teaspoons *kudzu*, dissolved in ¼ cup cold water

Heat the oil in a wok or skillet and sauté the onion and carrot over low heat for 5 minutes.

Add the stock, soy sauce, apple juice, and vinegar and bring to a boil. Reduce the heat and simmer gently for 3 minutes.

Taste and adjust the balance of apple juice and vinegar to taste. Add salt, if needed. Stir in the dissolved *kudzu* and stir until the sauce thickens.

Variations

- Add pieces of fresh pineapple for a tropical touch.
- Add sweet corn kernels and strips of red bell pepper.

Tomato-less Sauce

Yield: 4 servings

This recipe was created in 1970 by Mimi Gevaert, a member of the family that founded Lima Foods in Belgium, Europe's first macrobiotic food processors. She was a great enthusiast for Hokkaido pumpkins (Japanese pumpkins, bred from the original New England pumpkins brought to Japan by Commodore Perry in the nineteenth century). After enjoying them in Belgium, we brought seed back to the U.K. and enjoyed the first harvest in 1971. If you don't want to use tomatoes, Mimi's recipe comes as close to the flavor and texture of a tomato sauce as you can get.

2 onions, finely chopped
4 garlic cloves, chopped
3 tablespoons vegetable oil
1 carrot, finely grated
2 celery ribs, finely chopped
3 tablespoons soy sauce
2 tablespoons apple cider vinegar
3 tablespoons apple juice concentrate
1 cup vegetable stock or water
2 cups puréed pumpkin
1 small beet, boiled and puréed
½ teaspoon ground cinnamon
Tiny pinch of ground cloves
½ teaspoon black pepper
¼ teaspoon ground allspice

In a large saucepan or wok, sauté the onions and garlic in the oil until translucent. Add the carrot and celery and cook for 3 to 4 minutes. Add all of the remaining ingredients, reduce the heat to low, and simmer gently for 20 minutes.

Note: Needless to say, this recipe is also delicious served over pasta.

Sesame Sauce

Yield: 4 servings

This sauce had its beginnings in a simple dining concept: take one bowl of brown rice, sprinkle with soy sauce, pour tahini over, mix well, and eat. For those not very adept with chopsticks, this is a foolproof way to get the food from the bowl to the mouth—you just stab the rice, and it sticks to every available bit of chopstick!

In general, when tahini is used, we recommend that you use the white, hulled sesame purée. Although brown tahini is more of a whole food, the skin of the seed lends an earthy taste that can spoil this recipe.

10 tablespoons light tahini sesame cream
3 tablespoons soy sauce
2 cups vegetable stock or water

In a saucepan, mix the tahini, soy sauce, and stock together and cook over low heat for 5 minutes. The mixture should have a creamy consistency.

Add more water, if necessary, to achieve a creamy sauce.

Variation

- Add a pinch of grated lemon or orange zest for a zingy flavor.

Tamari Sauce

Yield: 4 servings

You can substitute shoyu *or other soy sauce for tamari in this recipe. This sauce goes particularly well with green vegetables.*

¼ cup plus 1 tablespoon tamari soy sauce
2½ tablespoons roasted (dark) sesame oil
¼ cup vegetable stock or water
1 tablespoon *kudzu*, dissolved in ¼ cup cold water

In a small saucepan, combine the tamari and oil and bring to a boil. Add the stock and boil for 3 minutes.

Add the dissolved *kudzu* to the boiling liquid, and stir constantly until the sauce thickens.

Mushroom Sauce

Yield: 2 servings

Mushrooms are a flavor enhancer because of their content of glutamic acid proteins. This sauce brings out their full flavor.

½ cup chopped mushrooms
1 onion, finely chopped
3 tablespoons olive oil
3 tablespoons whole wheat flour
1 cup vegetable stock, soy milk, or water
2 teaspoons soy sauce (optional)

In a skillet, sauté the mushrooms and onion in the oil for 5 minutes over low heat.

Add the flour and cook, stirring continuously, for 3 to 4 minutes, or until flour starts to give off a nutty, toasted smell.

Slowly add the stock, stirring constantly to prevent lumps from forming. Season with the soy sauce or salt to taste.

Serve over warm brown rice.

Pesto Sauce

Yield: 3 to 4 servings

Although pesto is a natural for pasta, it also goes well with brown rice.

    1 large bunch fresh basil
    4 garlic cloves
    ½ teaspoon sea salt
    ½ cup pine nuts
    ½ cup crumbled tofu
    ¼ cup plus 1 tablespoon olive oil

Remove the stems and pound the basil leaves in a mortar with the garlic, salt, and pine nuts. Add the tofu and blend well.

When the pesto is thick, add the olive oil a little at a time, stirring constantly.

The sauce should not be cooked. If you do not have a mortar and pestle, you can use a blender. Do not blend for long spells; use short bursts to keep the purée from becoming too smooth.

Cauliflower Sauce

Yield: 4 servings

When the cauliflower florets break up in this sauce, they give it a sweet aroma and a slightly grainy texture.

1 small cauliflower, whole
2 onions, chopped
¼ cup plus 1 tablespoon olive oil
3 tablespoons whole wheat flour
½ teaspoon sea salt
1 teaspoon soy sauce

Cook the cauliflower in boiling water for 10 minutes, or until soft. Drain, reserving 3½ cups of the cooking liquid. Set aside.

In a deep skillet, sauté the onions in the olive oil until translucent.

Add the flour, and cook, stirring constantly, for 2 to 3 minutes.

Add the cauliflower stock and stir to prevent lumps forming. Break up the cauliflower, and add it to the sauce. Season with the salt and soy sauce, turn down to a gentle heat, and simmer for 5 minutes.

Serve over warm brown rice.

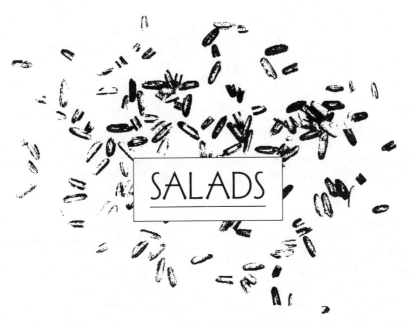

SALADS

Brown rice makes a perfect salad ingredient. From just a few grains sprinkled into a tossed salad to salads that consist of cooked room-temperature brown rice studded with a few piquant vegetables, brown rice lends itself to all sorts of cold and raw combinations.

Brown Rice and Vegetable Salad with Baked Beans

Yield: 6 servings

The baked beans in this recipe should be made with navy beans, not soybeans or pinto beans, which do not work as well.

Salad
cooked brown rice
1 (15-ounce) can sugar-free
   baked beans
3 scallions, thinly sliced
2 celery ribs, thinly sliced
½ red bell pepper, thinly
   sliced

Dressing
¼ cup plus 1 tablespoon
   olive oil
3 tablespoons cider vinegar
2 garlic cloves, crushed
1 teaspoon prepared mustard
Sea salt
Pepper

Garnish
¼ cup toasted,
   chopped almonds

In a bowl, combine the brown rice, beans, and vegetables.

Combine all of the dressing ingredients and shake together in a jar.

Pour the dressing over the salad, and fold in. Top with the almonds. Serve at once.

Muhammad's Chick-Pea Salad

Yield: 4 servings

This recipe was given to me by a friend's gardener in Tangier. I have varied the original by leaving out the copious amounts of cumin that Moroccans use with just about everything. However, you may find that a teaspoon or two of ground cumin makes an interesting addition.

Salad
- 1 pound green beans, sliced
- 2 cups cooked chick-peas
- 1 cup cooked brown rice
- 2 onions, sliced into rings

Vinaigrette
- ½ cup roasted (dark) sesame oil
- ¼ cup brown rice vinegar
- 2 garlic cloves, crushed
- 1 teaspoon prepared mustard
- 2 teaspoons soy sauce
- 2 teaspoons grated fresh ginger
- 1 tablespoon apple juice concentrate
- Sea salt
- Black pepper

Cook the green beans in boiling water until they are just tender, about 5 minutes. Drain and allow to cool.

In a bowl, combine beans, chick-peas, rice, and onions.

Combine all of the vinaigrette ingredients and shake together in a jar.

Pour the vinaigrette over the salad and toss to blend. Serve at once.

Salade de Puy

Yield: 4 servings

The tiny lentils de Puy, from Southern France, are unequalled in flavor so choose these small blue-green lentils if available. You can also use brown lentils or precooked lentils from cans or jars.

Dressing
½ cup olive oil
¼ cup apple cider vinegar
3 garlic cloves, crushed
1 teaspoon prepared mustard
Pinch of ground coriander
Sea salt

Salad
1 cup cooked lentils
1 cup cooked brown rice
½ cup sliced mushrooms
½ cup sliced scallions
½ green bell pepper, chopped
2 tablespoons toasted or raw pine nuts
½ cup peeled, seeded, and diced cucumber
¼ cup chopped parsley

Combine all of the dressing ingredients in a jar and shake well.

Warm the lentils and rice in a steamer.

Place the lentils and rice in a bowl and pour the dressing over them. Let stand for 15 minutes.

Add all of the remaining ingredients, blend well, and serve. (The dressing should have time to penetrate the lentils and rice without wilting the rest of the ingredients.)

Sunny Rice Salad

Yield: 4 servings

The sunflower seeds or pine nuts make all the difference in this salad. Toast them lightly for extra flavor and crunchiness.

Dressing
⅔ cup olive oil
¼ cup apple cider vinegar
2 garlic cloves, crushed
1 teaspoon prepared mustard
1 teaspoon black pepper
1 tablespoon lemon juice

Salad
3 cups cooked brown rice
½ red bell pepper, chopped
2 celery ribs, sliced
½ cup sunflower seeds or
  pine nuts

Combine all of the salad ingredients in a bowl.

Combine all of the dressing ingredients in a jar and shake well.

Pour the dressing over the salad and toss to coat.

Almond and Rice Salad

Yield: 4 servings

The almonds in this salad should be toasted thoroughly to get their full flavor. Sample them after they've cooked for 20 minutes, and if they aren't browned inside, leave them in a bit longer.

1 cup almonds
3 cups cooked brown rice
¼ teaspoon curry powder
½ cup olive oil
¼ cup rice vinegar
1 tablespoon lemon juice
1 teaspoon prepared mustard
½ cup chopped celery

Toast the almonds in a preheated 325° F oven for 20 minutes. Cool. Chop lightly.

Combine all of the remaining ingredients in a bowl. Blend in the almonds.

Serve immediately, or chill in the refrigerator.

Aduki Salad

Yield: 4 servings

Aduki beans develop a sweet flavor when they are cooked and then cooled. Make sure they don't break up too much when you are mixing the ingredients.

Dressing

¼ cup plus 1 tablespoon
  olive oil
2 tablespoons rice vinegar
2 garlic cloves, crushed
1 teaspoon prepared mustard
½ teaspoon sea salt
Pinch of black pepper
¼ cup chopped parsley
½ cup chopped celery
2 tablespoons chopped
  fresh dill

Salad

1 cup precooked cold aduki
  beans
1 cup cooked brown rice
6 scallions, chopped
½ cucumber, diced
½ cup diced daikon
Sea salt
Black pepper

Mix the dressing in a salad bowl (or whiz the ingredients in a food processor).

Add the beans and rice to the dressing and mix well. Let stand for 15 minutes.

Stir in the scallions, cucumber, and daikon. Season to taste with sea salt and black pepper. Serve right away.

Welsh Salad

Yield: 2 servings

Although the leek is Wales's national vegetable, the Welsh tend to boil leeks to death or use them as a base for soups. Raw, young leeks are milder than onions and give a pungency to this recipe.

Salad

2 leeks, well cleaned and
   finely shredded
3 celery ribs, finely chopped
2 carrots, peeled and grated
1 cup cooked brown rice

Dressing

3 tablespoons olive oil
1 tablespoon cider vinegar
1 teaspoon lemon juice
½ teaspoon prepared
   mustard
Sea salt and black pepper
Finely chopped parsley

Mix together the vegetables and rice in a salad bowl.

Mix the dressing ingredients and add to the salad. Toss to blend.

Serve with warm whole wheat bread.

Greek Hot Rice Salad

Yield: 2 servings

This quick and easy-to-prepare recipe comes from an old Mediterra-nean tradition; with only one fire and one cooking pot, you either cooked everything together as one dish or mixed raw ingredients with the hot.

½ teaspoon sea salt
1 teaspoon black pepper
1 onion, finely chopped
2 cups hot, cooked brown rice
¼ cup olive oil
2 tablespoons lemon juice
3 tablespoons chopped parsley

Garnish
Olives

Fold the salt, pepper, and onion into the hot rice.
Mix together the oil and lemon juice and pour over the rice. Sprinkle on the parsley and toss lightly.
Garnish with the olives, and serve while still warm.

Pink Rice Salad

Yield: 4 servings

This salad was an accident—I had no idea that beets would produce such a delightful and surprising hue. Pink food stands out, and the flavor of this salad is striking, too. It's a great recipe for parties and picnics.

1 beet
1 cup chopped celery
¼ cup chopped parsley
3 cups cooked brown rice
1 cup sliced daikon
½ cup olive oil
¼ cup apple cider vinegar
3 garlic cloves, crushed
1 teaspoon prepared mustard
2 teaspoons chopped dill or cilantro
Sea salt

Boil the beet in water to cover for 30 to 40 minutes until tender in the center. Allow to cool. Peel and coarsely grate the beet.

Combine all of the remaining ingredients. Add the grated beet and mix well until the salad turns the desired shade of pink. Serve at once.

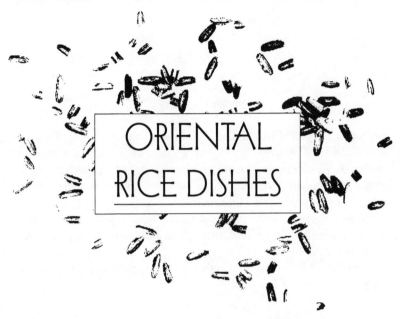

ORIENTAL RICE DISHES

Brown rice was the traditional staple diet of the countries of the East; not until the advent of colonialism and rice polishing did white rice become a popular food of "advanced" civilization. Even among Asian people in the West, consumption of brown rice is now rare, and a prejudice against it as the food of peasants will take a long time to disappear.

The pantheons of the early religions of many Eastern countries included a deity whose sole responsibility was to ensure a rice harvest of ample quantity and good quality, and perhaps also to ensure successful preparation of some of the recipes listed here.

Sushi

Yield: 1 serving

Sushi is a delightful way to combine brown rice and vegetables with the goodness of seaweed. Sea vegetables are rich in iodine, a mineral vital to the formation of thyroxine, the hormone that regulates the speed of the metabolism. No seaweed = no thyroxine = no energy—no matter how much coffee you drink.

To be successful with sushi you should have a sushi mat—a mat made of bamboo strips and string that holds everything in place while you roll it up.

For sushi it is best to have softer rice, so cook the rice with 1¾ to 2 parts of water to 1 part of rice.

1 sheet nori seaweed
1 cup cooked brown rice
Vegetables for filling, such as grated daikon, strips
     of tempeh (smoked or natural), strips of *takuan*
     radish pickle, strips of parboiled carrot, radish, or
     greens. A little umeboshi paste gives it bite, and
     so does a bit of sliced pickled ginger. Sometimes
     we just set out all the makings and let each per-
     son make his or her own combination.

Toast the nori seaweed by waving the sheet gently above a low flame—the color will change to green, and the sheet will crisp slightly.

Place the sheet of nori on a sushi mat.

Spread the rice evenly across the nori, leaving a ½-inch margin on all 4 sides.

Arrange an inch-wide stripe of vegetables about an inch from the bottom of the mat. With wet fingers and using the mat to keep things steady, roll the nori sheet up from the bottom, holding it firm. Use your wet fingers to dampen the top edge and help the nori stick together.

Cut the roll into 1-inch lengths with a very sharp knife, wetting the blade each time to prevent it from sticking and tearing the sushi.

Serve at once, or store covered for a few hours in the refrigerator.

Sushi Dip

Yield: 4 servings

Sushi is delicious with the following dip. Have a tissue ready for when your eyes water!

1 teaspoon wasabi horseradish powder
½ teaspoon water
1 tablespoon mirin (optional)
¼ cup soy sauce

Moisten the wasabi powder with the water and stir to form a paste. Combine the mirin and soy sauce.

Dissolve the wasabi paste in the soy/mirin mixture to achieve the desired degree of pungency.

Dip both ends of the sushi in the sauce and consume.

Can be stored in a jar in the refrigerator if not required until later.

Rice Balls

Yield: 2 servings (6–9 balls)

For traveling, when you don't know what food is going to be available, rice balls are the ideal companion. They will last several days, especially if you put a bit of umeboshi plum in the center. The rice you use has to be soft enough to stick together, ideally a short-grain variety. The finished rice ball should be a bit smaller than a tennis ball. They may sound bland, but when you've been away from decent food for a day or two, they can be your only link with reality.

3 sheets nori seaweed
3 cups soft-cooked short-grain brown rice
2 umeboshi plums, pitted and cut into quarters

Wave the nori sheets over a gentle flame for a few seconds; the color will turn from black to green, and the sheets will become crisper.

Fold the nori sheet in half, and tear into 2 pieces. Put these 2 pieces together, fold in half again, and tear to get 4 pieces.

Form a handful of rice into a ball. Put a piece of the umeboshi plum in the middle, and re-shape into a ball.

With wet fingers, pat enough sheets of nori around the ball to fully cover. (You may need only two pieces, depending on the size of the ball.)

Can be stored in an airtight container or in foil.

Variation

• You can tuck pieces of pickled daikon radish (*takuan*), pickled barley, or other condiments inside the rice ball.

Crispy Rice Balls

Yield: 2 servings (8 balls)

Fried rice balls are less portable and long-lived than nori-covered rice balls but are a good way of adding interest to leftover rice. They keep well wrapped in foil or plastic wrap.

2 cups cooked brown rice
2 umeboshi plums, pitted and cut into quarters
Vegetable oil
1 cup seasoned bread crumbs (page 13)

Form rice balls slightly larger than a ping-pong ball, with umeboshi plum in the middle as in the Rice Balls recipe (on the preceding page).

Roll the balls in seasoned bread crumbs, then shallow-fry in 1 inch of oil over medium heat until golden, turning once.

Drain on a cooling rack or paper towels.

Monk-Style Rice and Vegetables

Yield: 4 servings

This recipe gets its name from the vegetarian Zen Buddhist monks, who traditionally ate brown rice and vegetables as their main diet. The kudzu *holds together the vegetables and carries their combined flavors throughout the sauce. If you cannot obtain all of the vegetables, don't worry; substitute any vegetables you like. The principle is the same.*

1 onion, chopped
2 garlic cloves, sliced
2 tablespoons sesame oil
½ cup bean sprouts
½ cup black fungus mushrooms, soaked in water for 30 minutes
½ cup sliced shiitake mushrooms
1 carrot, sliced
½ cup finely sliced bamboo shoots

1 cup snow peas
1½ cups vegetable stock or water
2 tablespoons soy sauce
1 tablespoon apple juice concentrate
1 tablespoon *kudzu*, dissolved in ½ cup cold water
3 cups cooked brown rice

In a wok, sauté the onion and garlic in the sesame oil until golden, about 5 minutes.

Add all of the vegetables and mushrooms and stir-fry for 5 minutes.

Add the stock, the apple juice, and soy sauce, and simmer for 2 minutes.

Add the dissolved *kudzu* to the vegetable mixture, and cook, stirring constantly, until it thickens.

Serve straight away, hot, over the brown rice.

Pilau Rice

Yield: 4 servings

The turmeric in this recipe gives the dish a golden yellow color and a distinctive aroma.

2 onions, halved and sliced
3 tablespoons vegetable oil
1 cup frozen peas
½ teaspoon curry powder
10 black peppercorns
3 whole cloves
½ teaspoon turmeric powder
1½ cups grated fresh coconut
½ teaspoon sea salt
½ cup chopped, toasted almonds
½ cup chopped, toasted cashews
3 cups cooked brown rice

In a skillet, sauté the onions in the oil until golden, about 5 minutes.

Add all of the remaining ingredients and blend well. Stir in ¼ cup water. Cover and simmer for 4 minutes, or until the water is absorbed.

Remove the cloves and serve immediately.

Cauliflower Pilau

Yield: 4 servings

Cauliflower is rich in lignin, a type of fiber associated with woody plants. It adds a healthy as well as a flavorful dimension to this recipe.

2 cups cauliflower florets
Sea salt
Black pepper
3 tablespoons vegetable oil
1 onion, chopped
6 garlic cloves, chopped
½ teaspoon ground cinnamon
1 teaspoon grated fresh ginger
1 teaspoon ground cumin
Soy sauce
3 cups cooked brown rice

Sprinkle the cauliflower florets with salt and pepper. In a wok or skillet, fry the florets in the oil until they begin to turn golden and crisp at the edges. Remove from the pan.

Add the onion and garlic to the pan and sauté with the spices until translucent.

Return the cauliflower to the pan, along with all of the other ingredients. Mix well.

Spicy Rice

Yield: 4 servings

Sweet, milky, nutty, and spicy—this main course is a real luxury.

1 onion, finely chopped
½ cup cashew nuts
¼ cup grated coconut
¾ teaspoon fennel seeds
½ teaspoon poppy seeds
½ teaspoon mustard seeds
½ teaspoon ground cumin
½ teaspoon ground turmeric
3 tablespoons vegetable oil
3 cups cooked brown rice
½ cup raisins
¼ cup vegetable stock or water

In a skillet or saucepan, sauté the onion, cashews, coconut, seeds, cumin, and turmeric in the oil until the onions are translucent and golden, about 5 minutes.

Stir in the brown rice and raisins, and mix thoroughly. Pour the stock over the mixture. Cover and simmer for 5 minutes, or until the stock is absorbed. Serve immediately.

Tom Kha Tofu

Yield: 6 servings

*On our honeymoon my new wife and I attended the Thai Cookery
School at the Oriental Hotel in Bangkok. Thailand is a Buddhist
country and has a long history of vegetarian diet, based around
abundant vegetables and two main kinds of rice: the fragrant (i.e.
long-grain) rice of the north, and the sticky, blackish-purple rice of
the lowlands. Eating with sticky rice is a simple proposition: you
just grab a piece between your thumb and as many fingers as you
need to hold it together, and push it into whatever item on the table
appeals to you. The thumb moves out to squeeze on a piece of solid
food, while the rice soaks up some sauce. The whole thing is then
deftly conveyed to the mouth.*

*In modern Thailand, a spoon in the right hand and a fork in the
left replace bare hands.*

*The Buddhist disdain for killing animals has been sidestepped.
Thai Buddhists, reluctant to kill, get their Muslim neighbors to do
the slaughtering, and then eat the result with a clear conscience. As
our teacher said on the first day of the course: "If you are vegetarian and want to cook Thai-style, forget it." However, the principles
of cuisine are the same, with or without meat, and we successfully
adapted many recipes for vegetarian use—and mastered the art of
carving a tomato into a creditable imitation of a rose!*

*The recipe that follows is worth the effort and gets easier with
repetition. The original is called* Tom Kha Ghai *(Tom = soup, Kha
= galangal or Thai ginger, Ghai = chicken), but we substitute tofu
for chicken. It also is made with* prik nam, *a very hot small pepper. Like all peppers and capsicums, this is an imported nightshade,
brought from Brazil by Portuguese traders in the seventeenth century. Before then the Thais used green peppercorns exclusively for a
hot taste, as did everyone else in Asia. As green peppercorns are rich*

105

in chromium (of which most of us are deficient in this sugar-addicted age), we prefer them in place of hot peppers. We have not included tom pla, the fish sauce that is the omnipresent flavor enhancer of Thai cuisine. If you don't mind a little fermented fish, add some to taste. Thai spices freeze well, so if you have more green peppercorns or Kaffir lime leaf than you need, keep them in a container in the freezer. I use an ice cube tray to make cubes of chopped lemongrass or Thai ginger, a quick way of having these awkward-to-prepare herbs readily at hand.

5 shallots or 1 large onion, finely chopped
5 garlic cloves, finely chopped
¼ cup vegetable oil
½ cup chopped galangal (Thai ginger, *kha)*
¼ cup chopped lemongrass
1 tablespoon chopped fresh green peppercorns
1 tablespoon chopped cilantro (coriander) roots
4 cups frozen or canned unsweetened coconut milk
2 cups frozen peas
1 cup diced carrots
1½ cups cubed tofu
2 tablespoons lime juice or lemon juice
1 cup chopped cilantro (coriander) leaves
1 tablespoon finely sliced Kaffir lime leaf
2 teaspoons soy sauce
1 teaspoon sea salt
6 cups cooked brown rice

In a wok, sauté the shallots and garlic in the oil until light golden, about 5 minutes.

Add the galangal, lemongrass, green peppercorns, and cilantro roots, and stir-fry for 3 minutes.

Add the coconut milk, and bring to a boil. Reduce the heat and simmer for 3 minutes.

Add the peas, carrots, and tofu and simmer for 5 or 6 minutes, or until the vegetables are barely cooked.

Stir in the lime juice, cilantro leaves, and Kaffir lime leaf. Season with the soy sauce and sea salt to taste. Remove from the heat. Serve immediately in a large bowl.

On each plate, make a well of the cooked brown rice, and ladle the soup into the well.

Leftovers store well in a bowl or airtight container.

Variations

- If you can't find galangal (Thai ginger), use ordinary ginger, but halve the quantity. Use precooked chick-peas in place of the tofu, or any other vegetables. Chopped greens are particularly good.

- If you prefer, use soy milk in place of coconut milk. The basic soup lends itself to infinite interpretations based on seasonal availability of vegetables and your own creative input.

Abargoo Rice

Yield: 4 servings

In 1965 I was hitchhiking eastward across southern Iran, when I was unexpectedly stranded at nightfall with no sign of civilization, except a mud wall a few hundred yards off the road to the right. A door opened in the wall and about 20 people came running ominously towards me, only to insist that I be the guest of the village for the night. How could I refuse?

That evening it seemed as though everybody in the village passed through the house I was in, as they stayed up late into the evening, playing drums and flutes and eating unleavened bread, fried eggs, and a rice dish studded with raisins and nuts.

The next morning they all came down to the road with me to block the first truck that came by and insist that the driver give me a ride to Yazd, the next town down the road from their village of Abargoo.

½ cup pine nuts
½ cup chopped almonds
¼ cup olive oil (they used goat's milk butter)
3 cups long-grain brown rice
½ cup raisins

½ cup water
½ teaspoon ground cinnamon
½ teaspoon black pepper
½ teaspoon sea salt
Tiny pinch of ground cloves

In a skillet or wok, fry the pine nuts and almonds in the oil until lightly browned, no more than 5 minutes; do not let them burn.

Add all of the remaining ingredients. Cover and simmer for 2 minutes.

Serve hot, lukewarm, or cold.

My Fava Rice Thing

Yield: 4 servings

Broad beans, or fava beans, are the first vegetables to ripen in the early summer, and in the Middle East people seem to eat nothing else when they are in season. Fresh or frozen lima beans can be used as well.

3 tablespoons olive oil
1 onion, chopped
4 garlic cloves, chopped
2 cups fresh or frozen broad (fava) beans
¼ teaspoon sea salt
½ teaspoon black pepper
1 teaspoon ground coriander
½ teaspoon ground cumin
¼ cup lemon juice
1 cup water
3 cups cooked brown rice

Garnish
Parsley

In a skillet, heat the oil and sauté the onion and garlic until golden.

Add the broad beans and sauté for another 3 minutes.

Add the salt, pepper, spices, lemon juice, and water, and bring to a boil. Reduce the heat and simmer for 5 minutes.

Stir in the rice. Cover, and cook until the water is absorbed.

Serve garnished with parsley.

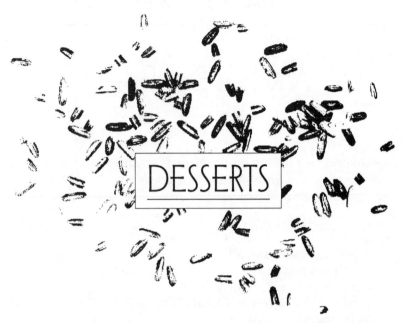

DESSERTS

Most of the brown rice grain is starch, a complex carbohydrate. (This is the food for the plant that the grain would have been, if it hadn't become food for you instead.)

When you chew rice, your saliva enzymes start to turn the brown rice starch into complex chains of glucose molecules called maltodextrins. These will in turn break down into shorter chains of glucose called maltose, and then into glucose, which is the basic sugar fuel of the human metabolism. Good health depends on a stable level of blood glucose. Eating sugar raises blood sugar sharply, and stressfully, as the metabolism struggles to bring it back down to normal. Usually, it comes down too far, leading to hunger, apathy, fatigue, and a consequent craving for sweet food to quickly raise the blood sugar back to normal.

A healthy diet is one in which you are in control, and in which you are not driven by irrational hunger that leads to overeating, obesity, and strain on the digestive system. This means keeping sugar consumption to a minimum, and eating foods that are digested more slowly, thereby keeping the blood sugar level in equilibrium. The ideal desserts are those that satisfy the desire for sweetness without containing a lot of quickly digested simple sugars.

Grain syrups, such as brown rice syrup and barley malt syrup, provide slower-burning maltose and maltodextrins, and these are preferred sweeteners. Apple juice concentrate is high in fructose, which is more slowly absorbed, so this is also a desirable sweetener. Grape juice concentrate is almost pure glucose, so it raises blood sugar levels too quickly and is not used in these recipes.

Rice Pudding

Yield: 4 servings

When we first introduced brown rice in our London restaurant and shop, we always used the more yang, short-grain brown rice. For many of our customers this presented a psychological barrier; they inextricably linked short-grain rice with the taste of the cinnamon, cream, and eggs that go into a traditional rice pudding, and couldn't relate to the same type of rice being used with vegetables.

This recipe excludes eggs and uses soy milk instead of dairy milk, but still perfectly captures the essence of the standard pudding. It's also delicious made with Basmati rice.

3 cups cooked brown rice
3 cups soy milk
½ teaspoon salt
½ teaspoon vanilla extract
1 teaspoon grated lemon zest
1 teaspoon ground cinnamon
¼ cup rice syrup or barley malt

In a saucepan or double boiler, combine all of the ingredients and bring to a boil. Stir frequently over low heat or simmering water, until the pudding becomes thick and creamy.

Serve the pudding hot. It is delicious topped with a spoonful of fruit-juice–sweetened jam.

Baked Rice Pudding

Yield: 4 servings

Although baked rice puddings usually call for eggs, this recipe comes out lighter and more digestible without them.

3 cups cooked brown rice
2 cups soy milk
Pinch of salt
¼ cup malt or grain syrup
1 teaspoon vanilla extract
1 teaspoon grated lemon zest
½ cup raisins

Preheat the oven to 325° F. Oil a medium-sized, deep baking dish.

In a bowl, combine all of the ingredients. The mixture should be runny enough that there is a thin layer of liquid on the surface.

Place the mixture in the prepared baking dish. Cover and bake for 40 to 50 minutes, until the top is browned.

Rice Smoothies

Yield: 4 servings

This is a nice way to get a smooth, cool, fruity, creamy summer snack that doesn't wreak havoc with your waistline or your digestion.

1 cup cooked brown rice
2 cups soy milk
1 cup fruit-juice–sweetened jam

Combine all of the ingredients in a blender and blend until smooth. The mixture should be just pourable.
Refrigerate before serving.

Moholobia

Yield: 4 servings

In the Levant, people eat this dessert as a popular between-meal snack, served in little glass bowls.

2 cups cooked brown rice
2 cups soy milk
½ teaspoon sea salt
½ teaspoon vanilla extract
1 teaspoon grated lemon zest
¼ cup rice syrup or barley malt
1 tablespoon rosewater*

Garnish
3 tablespoons chopped pistachio nuts

In a saucepan or double boiler, combine all of the ingredients and bring to a boil. Stir frequently over a low heat or simmering water, until the pudding becomes thick and creamy.

Divide among 4 glass bowls. Sprinkle with the chopped pistachio nuts to garnish.

Refrigerate for at least 1 hour and serve cold. (The pudding does not come out as firm as it would if made with cow's milk.)

* If you can't get rosewater, use rose petals from a fragrant rose, ideally a damask rose, and steep them in a little boiling water for 30 minutes before use. Leave the rose petals in if you wish; like many flowers, they are completely edible. (Make sure that the roses have not been sprayed with any toxic chemicals.)

Tropical Pudding

Yield: 4 servings

The lime is the essential flavor ingredient in this recipe. If you can use a little finely chopped Kaffir lime leaf (from a Thai grocer), all the better.

Grated zest and juice of 1 lime
2 cups cooked brown rice
¼ teaspoon sea salt
3 tablespoons rice syrup
2 cups unsweetened coconut milk
2 cups chopped pineapple or mangoes

In a saucepan, combine the lime zest, rice, salt, syrup, and coconut milk, and bring to a boil. Reduce the heat and simmer gently, stirring occasionally, until thick.

Add the chopped fruit and lime juice, and cook, stirring, for 3 minutes. Serve hot.

BROWN RICE AND FASTING

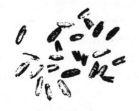

The main factor that has led to the widespread consumption of brown rice is the spread of the macrobiotic way of eating in the United States and Europe in the past two decades. The macrobiotic philosophy, based on the dialectical principle of yin and yang, enables you to judge the correct balance of your diet without needing to memorize or frequently refer to calorie charts or lists of mineral and vitamin contents of food. It does this by putting a balanced food—brown rice—at the heart of your diet. As long as your diet is based upon a principal food such as whole-grain rice, you can eat other foods without upsetting the overall balance.

The macrobiotic diet has a positive goal, seeking to maximize your physical, mental, and spiritual potential by maintaining a body that, thanks to good diet and regular activity, is functioning at the peak of its capabilities. However, the transition from eating a conventional diet is helped by a period of fasting, when you can get in tune with your body and break the ingrained dietary habits that control your appetite. Fasting also gives your digestive organs a break and strengthens your immune system.

As a means of enabling the body to cleanse and restore itself, George Ohsawa, the founder of modern macrobiotic philosophy, introduced Diet Number Seven, a seven-day diet based solely on brown rice. Much disease originates in intestinal malfunction, which results in poor blood quality. By restoring intestinal motility and effectiveness, the brown rice diet can ameliorate many chronic conditions.

After an initial difficult period, going without food is not a very distressing process. With practice, fasting becomes much easier, and fast days and other variations on fasting themes are a traditional feature of most of the world's cultures and religions.

A fast using brown rice is the easiest way to enjoy fasting's benefits without having to do without food entirely. It also cultivates an awareness and appreciation of the advantages of careful chewing, enhances one's enjoyment of the flavor of rice, and leads to a greater understanding of the role of brown rice and other whole cereals in balancing one's nutrition. With crash starvation diets, the metabolism slows down, and when you start to eat normally again, your body puts on weight in anticipation of the next period of starvation. With a brown rice diet, you are training yourself to need less and to get the most out of the food you eat.

It is not advisable to eat a diet based exclusively on brown rice for more than a few days at the outset, and one should not exceed a week on the diet without good reason, preferably with medical consultation.

A brown rice fast can include small amounts of the following foods: sea salt used in preparation of the rice, gomasio sesame salt, tamari soy sauce, and tahini sesame seed cream. Gomasio is made by combining 16 parts of lightly toasted sesame seeds with 1 part of sea salt and grinding them together, either with a pestle in a mortar or with a peppermill. Readymade gomasios are available from many natural food shops, but they lack the flavor of the freshly made condiment. You may be quite thirsty at first. Drinks should be limited to green tea, mineral water, and herbal teas.

A rice gruel can be made by adding water to cooked rice to the desired consistency. Lightly seasoned with soy sauce or gomasio, this gruel is an ideal way of getting invalids to take food, as well as being a variation to include in a brown rice fast.

PREPARING BROWN RICE FOR FASTING

Sesame Rice

Lightly toast whole sesame seeds in a dry frying pan. Stir into the rice, adding about 1 tablespoon of seeds per cupful of cooked rice.

Umeboshi Rice

Pit a few umeboshi plums and break the plum flesh into 4 to 5 pieces. Scatter them over the rice before cooking. (Use no salt in preparing this rice, as there is an adequate amount in the plum.)

Miso Rice

Dissolve 1 teaspoon miso soybean paste in each cupful of water used in preparing the rice. Boil the rice in the usual way. If you are pressure-cooking the rice, use one-third less miso per cupful of water. Miso, tamari, or *shoyu* sauce can also be added after cooking the rice, but the flavor infuses the grains if added before cooking.

Herb Rice

You may wish to include a specific herb in your diet such as parsley, mugwort, or thyme. When the rice is cooked, stir in a teaspoonful or so of the herb and allow to stand for another 10 minutes. The steam and heat of the rice will draw out the herbal flavors. Adding herbs before cooking will lead to overcooking the herbs and destroying their flavor.

Raw Rice

For intestinal problems, and particularly for purging intestinal parasites, a handful of raw rice eaten as the first food of the day—and chewed very thoroughly—can be very effective. Raw food is always beneficial to the digestive system as it is assimilated farther down the intestines than cooked food, and raw grains in small quantities can be very effective in restoring tone and vitality to this important organ.

INDEX

NOTE: Recipe titles are capitalized

Abargoo Rice, 108
aduki beans, 8; Aduki Rice, 46;
  Aduki Salad, 91; Rice and Peas, 47
alcohol, 5
Almond and Rice Salad, 90
Almond Sauce, 76
almonds, 24, 86, 102, 108
amino acids, 7, 18
anemia, 50
appetite, 6, 13–14
arrowroot, 36
Autumn Risotto, 53

Bean Sprout and Rice Patties, 71
beans, aduki, 8, 46, 47, 91; baked,
  86; black, 8; with brown rice,
  7–8; chick-pea, 8, 35, 87; chili, 7;
  fava, 8, 109; green, 87; lentils,
  7–8, 88; preparing, 7–8; sprouts,
  40, 71, 77, 101
Béchamel Sauce, Mock, 55, 70, 74;
  Mustard, 27, 74; Wasabi, 75
Belizian Brown Rice Mix-it-up, 48–
  49
Boiled Brown Rice, 22
bran, 2, 20
bread, 7; crumbs, seasoned, 13, 54,
  57, 61, 66, 100
breakfast foods, Miso Soup, 40–41;
  Rice Cream Cereal, 29
brown rice, 1–2. *See also* rice; with

beans, 7–8; complimentary foods,
  7–13; cooking methods, 20–21;
  for fasting, 117–120; reheating,
  25; with sea vegetables, 11; with
  soy foods, 9–10; syrup, 13, 41,
  111, 112, 115, 116; with
  vegetables, 8–9, 44; with wild
  vegetables, 11–12
brown rice recipes, Baked, 24;
  Boiled, 22; Chestnut Rice, 28;
  for fasting, 119–120; Gruel, 119;
  Hearty Brown Rice Soup, 35;
  Herb Rice, 119; Miso Rice, 119;
  Popped, 30; Pressure Cooked, 23;
  Raw Rice, 120; Rice Cream Cereal,
  29; Sesame Rice, 119; Steamed,
  25, 26; Umeboshi Rice, 119; with
  vegetables, 8–9, 43; Wheat and
  Rice, 27; with wild rice, 18
Brown Rice and Carrots, 44
Brown Rice and Peanut Butter Bake,
  72
Brown Rice and Peas, 47
Brown Rice and Vegetable Salad
  with Baked Beans, 86
Brown Rice Patties, 70
Brown Rice Tray *Kibbeh*, 68–69
buckwheat, roasted, 67

cabbage, 33, 53; greens, 50, 58
Cabbage Rolls, 64
Carrots and Brown Rice, 44
Cashew Risotto, 57

121

cashews, 57, 102, 104
casseroles, 52. *See also* patties;
    risottos; vegetables and brown
    rice; Baked Brown Rice, 24;
    Brown Rice Tray *Kibbeh*, 68–69;
    Cabbage Rolls, 64; Peanut Rice
    Supreme, 65; Stuffed Onions, 66;
    Stuffed Summer Squash, 67;
    Stuffed Vine Leaves, 62–63;
    Tempeh Casserole, 54–55
Cauliflower Rice, 103
Cauliflower Sauce, 84
Chestnut Rice, 28
chick-peas, 8, 35; Muhammad's
    Chick-Pea Salad, 87
coconut, 47, 49, 102, 104, 106, 116
Crispy Rice Balls, 100

dairy products, 5
desserts, 110–111; Baked Rice
    Pudding, 113; Moholobia, 115;
    Rice Pudding, 112; Rice
    Smoothies, 114; Tropical
    Pudding, 116
diet, 4, 8, 14, 117–120
Dill and Pea Béchamel Sauce, 75

fasting, 117–120
fats, 8, 11
flavor, garlic enhancing, 45;
    mushrooms enhancing, 33, 82;
    oils enhancing, 11; stocks
    enhancing, 31; vegetable
    preparation enhancing, 9;
    vegetable stock enhancing, 12–13,
    31; wild rice enhancing, 18
fruit, currants, 59; juice, 13, 41, 78,
    87, 111, 114, 116; raisins, 13, 59,
    104, 108, 113

Garlic and Rice Soup, 37
gomasio, 12, 118
grain syrups, 111
grape leaves, Stuffed Vine Leaves,
    62–63
Greek Hot Rice Salad, 93
greens, cabbage, 50, 58; chickweed,
    11; collard, 50; dandelion, 11, 50,
    58; endive, 50; kale, 50; mustard,

58, 60; radicchio, 50, 60; Rice and
    Greens, 50; in risottos, 58, 60;
    wild, 11–12

hazlenuts, 67
health, 4–6
Herb Rice, 119
herbs, 34, 50, 106. *See also* season-
    ings
hummus, 7

immune system, 50, 117

kitchen utensils, 14
kudzu, 36

leftovers recipes, Brown Rice Patties,
    70; Risotto in Salto, 61; Vegetable
    Sauce, 77
lemon, juice, 12, 38, 41, 50, 76, 89,
    92, 93, 106, 109; in Sesame
    Sauce, 80; zest, 38, 50, 57, 80,
    112, 113, 115, 116
Lemon Soup, Tangy, 38
lime, 106
lysine, 7, 18

macrobiotics, 1–2, 4–6, 117–119
malt, 13, 112, 113, 115
microwave, 25
miso purée, 9–10; genmai miso, 10,
    40
Miso Rice, 119
Miso Soup with Brown Rice, 40–41
Moholobia, 115
Muhammad's Chick-Pea Salad, 87
mushrooms, 33, 45, 66, 88, 101;
    Mushroom Sauce, 82; Mushrooms
    and Rice, 45
Mustard Béchamel Sauce, 74
My Fava Rice Thing, 109

nettles, 11; Nettle Soup, 42
nightshades, 5
nuts, pistachio, 60

oil, 10–11, 75
olives, Greek Hot Rice Salad, 93
organic food, 5, 8, 18–19, 44

Index

oriental rice dishes, 95; Abargoo Rice, 108; Cauliflower Rice, 103; Crispy Rice Balls, 100; Monk-Style Rice and Vegetables, 101; My Fava Rice Thing, 109; Pilau Rice, 102; Rice Balls, 99; Spicy Rice, 104; Sushi, 96–97; Sushi Dip, 98; Tom Kha Tofu, 105–107

pasta, 34, 79
patties, 52; Bean Sprout and Rice Patties, 71; Brown Rice Patties, 70; Risotto in Salto, 61
Pea and Dill Béchamel Sauce, 75
Peanut Butter and Brown Rice Bake, 72
Peanut Rice Supreme, 65
Peas and Rice, 47
Peas and Tarragon Rice, 51
pesticides, 5, 8, 44
Pesto Sauce, 83
pilafs, 25
Pilau Rice, 102
pita bread, 7
Popped Brown Rice, 30
Pressure-Cooked Brown Rice, 23
protein, 7, 33

Raw Rice, 120
rice. See also brown rice; basmati, 16, 112; black, 17; brown, 1–2; long grain, 16; medium grain, 16; organic farming methods, 18–19; parboiled (converted), 17–18; quick rice, 17; red, 16–17; short grain, 15, 112; sweet brown, 16; syrup, 41, 111, 112, 115, 116; varieties, 15–19; white, 2–3, 17, 18; wild, 18; wine (mirin), 12, 98
Rice Balls, 99
Rice Cream Cereal, 29
Rice Pudding, 31, 112
Rice Pudding, Baked, 113
Rice Smoothies, 114
Risi i Bisi, 56
Risotto in Salto, 61
risottos, 52; Autumn Risotto, 53; Cashew Risotto, 57; Italian, 15; Risi i Bisi, 56; Risotto in Salto, 61; Risoverde, 60; Spring Risotto, 58; Sunshine Risotto, 59
Risoverde, 60

salad dressings, 88, 89, 91, 92; vinaigrette, 87
Salade de Puy, 88
salads, 85; Aduki Salad, 91; Almond and Rice Salad, 90; Brown Rice and Vegetable Salad with Baked Beans, 86; Greek Hot Rice Salad, 93; Muhammad's Chick-Pea Salad, 87; Pink Rice Salad, 94; Salade de Puy, 88; Sunny Rice Salad, 89; Welsh Salad, 92
salt, for rice, 12, 20–21, 22
sauces, 73; Almond Sauce, 76; Cauliflower Sauce, 84; Dill and Pea Béchamel Sauce, 75; fish sauce, 12; Mock Béchamel Sauce, 27, 74; Mushroom Sauce, 82; Mustard Béchamel Sauce, 74; Pesto Sauce, 83; Sesame Sauce, 80; Sushi Dip, 98; Sweet and Sour Sauce, 78; Tamari Sauce, 81; for Tempeh Casserole, 54; Tomato-less Sauce, 79; Vegetable Sauce, 77; Wasabi Béchamel Sauce, 75
seasonings, allspice, 68; basil, 83; bonito flakes, 12; burdock root, 11; cilantro, 34, 94; cinnamon, 31, 49, 68, 103, 112; for color, 31; coriander, 31, 34, 109; cumin, 87, 103, 104, 109; curry, 31, 90, 102; dill, 50, 91, 94; fennel, 33, 50, 104; garlic, 33, 37, 45, 62, 64, 67, 79, 88, 101, 103, 106, 109; ginger, 50, 77, 87, 96, 103, 106; marjoram, 50, 67; mustard, 86–92, 94, 104; parsley, 33, 37, 50, 53, 57, 74, 91, 93, 94; pepper, 102, 106, 108, 109; for rice pudding, 31; saffron, 24, 31; salt, 12; seasoned bread crumbs, 13, 54, 57, 61, 66, 100; for stock, 34; thyme, 66; tumeric, 24, 31, 102, 104; wasabi, 50
seaweed, 11, 12; arame, 11; kombu, 11, 33, 46; nori, 11, 12, 35, 62,

96–97, 99; for Sushi, 96–97;
  wakame, 11, 41
seeds, 59, 104; pine nuts, 62, 68, 83,
  88, 89, 108; pumpkin, 30;
  sunflower, 30, 59, 70, 71, 89
seitan, 68–69
sesame, oil, 11, 40, 50, 65, 78, 81,
  87, 101; seeds, 12, 30, 44, 118;
  tahini, 80
Sesame Rice, 119
Sesame Sauce, 80
sleep, 6
soups, 32; Garlic and Rice Soup, 37;
  Hearty Brown Rice Soup, 35; Miso
  Soup with Brown Rice, 40–41;
  Nettle Soup, 42; Sweet Corn
  and Rice Soup, 39; Tangy Lemon
  Soup, 38; thickeners, 36; Tofu
  Islands, 36; Vegetable Stock,
  12–13, 31, 33–34
soy foods, 9–10; miso purée, 9–10;
  soy milk, 10, 56, 107, 112–115;
  tamari, 9, 24, 81; tempeh, 10, 78,
  96; tofu, 10
soy sauce (shoyu), 9, 12, 24
Spicy Rice, 104
Spring Risotto, 58
starch, 110
stir-fry, 9, 11
Stuffed Onions, 66
Stuffed Summer Squash, 67
sugar, 5, 13, 110–111
Sunshine Risotto, 59
Sushi, 96–97
Sushi Dip, 98
Sweet and Sour Sauce, 78
Sweet Corn and Rice Soup, 39

Tamari Sauce, 81
Tangy Lemon Soup, 38
Tarragon Rice and Peas, 51
tea, for rice stock, 31
Tempeh Casserole, 54–55
tempura, sauce for, 78
tofu, 10, 36, 38, 57, 65, 72; Brown
  Rice and Peanut Butter Bake, 72;
  sauce for, 78; Tom Kha Tofu,
  105–107

Tofu Islands, 36
Tom Kha Tofu, 105–107
Tomato-less Sauce, 79
Tropical Pudding, 116

umeboshi, in Rice Balls, 99, 100; in
  Sushi, 96; Umeboshi Rice, 119

vanilla, 112, 113, 115
Vegetable and Brown Rice Salad
  with Baked Beans, 86
Vegetable Sauce, 77
vegetable stock, 12–13, 31, 33–34
vegetables, added to rice, 24; beets,
  31, 79, 94; bell pepper, 88, 89;
  with brown rice, 8–9, 43–51;
  carrots, 92, 106; cauliflower, 50;
  celery, 33, 65, 79, 86, 90–92, 94;
  combining in stock, 33; corn, 7,
  39, 78; cucumber, 88, 91; daikon,
  91, 94, 96, 99; leeks, 33, 39, 58,
  92; onions, 33, 35, 37, 42, 48, 64,
  79, 84, 87, 101; peas, 54, 56, 60,
  101, 102, 106; plantain, 48;
  preparing, 9; pumpkin, 79; in
  sauces, 77; scallions, 50, 58, 70,
  86, 88, 91; spinach, 60; squash,
  53, 67; takuan pickle, 96; wild,
  11–12, 42
vegetarianism, 8, 105
vinaigrette, 87. *See also* salad
  dressings
vinegar, 12, 78, 79, 86–92, 94
vitamins, 2–3, 18, 50

wasabi, 50, 98
Wasabi Béchamel Sauce, 75
water, for boiled rice, 22; for
  pressure-cooked rice, 23; for salt-
  free rice, 21; stocks in place of,
  31, 34
Welsh Salad, 92
Wheat and Rice, 27
wheat (bulgur), in Brown Rice Tray
  Kibbeh, 68–69
wok, 14